KU-740-105

Hypertension

Commissioning Editor: Laurence Hunter
Development Editor: Clive Hewat
Project Manager: Frances Affleck
Designer: Erik Bigland
Illustrator: David Gardner

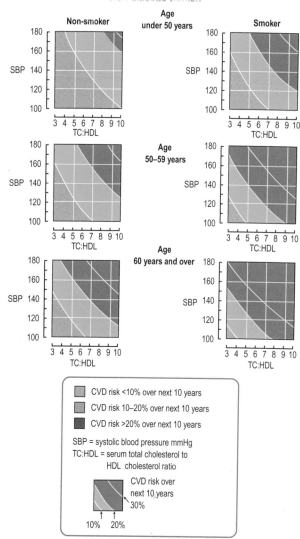

Cardiovascular Disease Risk Prediction Chart
Non-diabetic women

Non-smoker | Age under 50 years | **Smoker**

Age 50–59 years

Age 60 years and over

SBP (axis values: 100, 120, 140, 160, 180)
TC:HDL (axis values: 3 4 5 6 7 8 9 10)

CVD risk <10% over next 10 years
CVD risk 10–20% over next 10 years
CVD risk >20% over next 10 years

SBP = systolic blood pressure mmHg
TC:HDL = serum total cholesterol to
          HDL cholesterol ratio

CVD risk over
next 10 years
30%

10% 20%

Hypertension

Isla S. Mackenzie MBChB MRCP
Clinical Lecturer in Clinical Pharmacology,
University of Cambridge, Cambridge, UK

Ian B. Wilkinson MA DM MRCP
Lecturer in Clinical Pharmacology and Honorary
Consultant Physician, Addenbrooke's Hospital,
University of Cambridge, Cambridge, UK

John R. Cockcroft BSc (Hons) MB ChB FRCP
Professor and Honorary Consultant in
Cardiology, Wales Heart Research Institute,
University of Wales School of Medicine,
Cardiff, UK

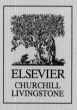

ELSEVIER
CHURCHILL
LIVINGSTONE

EDINBURGH LONDON NEW YORK OXFORD
PHILADELPHIA ST LOUIS SYDNEY TORONTO 2005

ELSEVIER
CHURCHILL
LIVINGSTONE

First published 2005

ISBN 0443074623

British Library Cataloguing in Publication Data
A catalogue record for this book is available from the British Library

Library of Congress Cataloging in Publication Data
A catalog record for this book is available from the Library of Congress

Notice
Medical knowledge is constantly changing. Standard safety precautions must be followed, but as new research and clinical experience broaden our knowledge, changes in treatment and drug therapy may become necessary or appropriate. Readers are advised to check the most current product information provided by the manufacturer of each drug to be administered to verify the recommended dose, the method and duration of administration, and contraindications. It is the responsibility of the practitioner, relying on experience and knowledge of the patient, to determine dosages and the best treatment for each individual patient. Neither the publisher nor the authors assume any liability for any injury and/or damage to persons or property arising from this publication.
The Publisher

Printed in China

CONTENTS

PREFACE

The first measurements of blood pressure were made in animals in the 18th century. However, it was some time later that blood pressure was measured in humans for the first time. Despite the development of the modern mercury sphygmomanometer around 100 years ago, the full clinical significance of high blood pressure or hypertension was only recognized after several years. Hypertension is now firmly established as a major modifiable cardiovascular risk factor.

The first truly effective and tolerable drug therapies for hypertension were the thiazide diuretics which were introduced in the 1950s. In 1971, Edward Freis was awarded the Albert Lasker prize for demonstrating the effectiveness of drug treatment in hypertension in terms of reducing cardiovascular events when arterial pressure is lowered to normal values. There is now a plethora of drug therapies available for treating hypertension, including most recently the calcium channel blockers, ACE inhibitors and angiotensin receptor antagonists. Interestingly, most outcome trials, with a few notable exceptions, have shown that it is the blood pressure reduction itself rather than the choice of antihypertensive agent that is most important in reducing cardiovascular risk.

In younger people with essential hypertension we are now perhaps approaching the maximum therapeutic benefits that can be achieved with current therapy. However, in most ageing Western societies, the boundaries between hypertension due to normal vascular ageing and that resulting from abnormal pathophysiology, are becoming increasingly blurred. Such arterial stiffening associated with age and disease has become a new and important therapeutic target in terms of blood pressure reduction and cardiovascular disease prevention in the elderly. Antihypertensive agents designed to prevent or reverse arterial stiffening are already being developed and look set to usher in yet another new and exciting area in the treatment of hypertension.

This book is written at a time when hypertension is, according to the World Health Organisation, the third highest cause of death and morbidity worldwide. Despite this, it is consistently under-diagnosed and under-treated in most developed countries. This book is therefore intended to provide an up-to-date review of evidence-based diagnosis and treatment of hypertension, including non-pharmacological intervention. We believe that such a book is timely, as due to the increased longevity of most modern populations the lifetime risk of developing hypertension of a normotensive individual who is currently 55 years old is 90%. This projected increase in the prevalence of hypertension should spur us on to redouble our efforts to improve the diagnosis and control of this major risk factor.

I. S. M

I. B. W

J. R. C

ACKNOWLEDGEMENTS

The authors would like to acknowledge Mrs Janet Usher and Mrs Angela Loveridge for secretarial assistance – and Professor Morris Brown, Dr Mark Gurnell and Dr Khin Swe Myint for help with clinical images.

ABBREVIATIONS

4S Scandinavian Simvastatin Survival Study

ABCD Appropriate Blood Pressure Control in Diabetes

ABPM ambulatory blood pressure monitoring

ACE angiotensin-converting enzyme

ACTH adrenocorticotrophic hormone

ALLHAT Antihypertensive and Lipid-Lowering Treatment to Prevent Heart Attack Trial

ALLHAT–LLT Antihypertensive and Lipid-Lowering Treatment to Prevent Heart Attack Trial – Lipid Lowering Trial

ASCOT–LLA Anglo-Scandinavian Cardiac Outcomes Trial–Lipid Lowering Arm

BHS British Hypertension Society

BMI body mass index

CAPP Captopril Prevention Project

CHD coronary heart disease

CT computerized tomography

DASH Dietary Approaches to Stop Hypertension

EUROPA European Trial on Reduction of Cardiac Events with Perindopril in Stable Coronary Artery Disease

FACET Fosinopril Versus Amlodipine Cardiovascular Events Randomized Trial

GEMINI Glycemic Events in Diabetes Mellitus: Carvedilol–Metoprolol Comparison in Hypertensives

HDL high-density lipoprotein

HELLP haemolysis, elevated liver enzymes and low platelets

HOPE Heart Outcomes Prevention Evaluation

HOT Hypertension Optimal Treatment

HPS Heart Protection Study

HYVET Hypertension in the Very Elderly Trial

INSIGHT International Nifedipine GITS Study: Intervention as a Goal in Hypertension Treatment

IRMA2 Irbesartan In Patients with Type 2 Diabetes and Microalbuminuria study

JNC 7 Seventh report of the Joint National Committee on Prevention, Detection, Evaluation, and Treatment of High Blood Pressure

LDL low-density lipoprotein

LIFE Losartan Intervention for Endpoint Reduction in Hypertension

MIBG ^{131}I-metaiodobenzylguanidine

MRC Medical Research Council

MRI magnetic resonance imaging

NHS National Health Service

NIDDM non-insulin-dependent diabetes mellitus

NORDIL Nordic Diltiazem Study

NSAID non-steroidal anti-inflammatory drug

PEACE Prevention of Events with Angiotensin Converting Enzyme Inhibition Trial

PRAISE Prospective Randomized Amlodipine Survival Evaluation

PROGRESS Perindopril Protection Against Recurrent Stroke Study

RENAAL Reduction of Endpoints in NIDDM with the Angiotensin II Antagonist Losartan

SHEP Systolic Hypertension in the Elderly Program

STOP Swedish Trial in Old Patients with Hypertension

STOP–2 Swedish Trial in Old Patients with Hypertension–2

UKPDS UK Prospective Diabetes Study

VLDL very low-density lipoprotein

WOSCOPS West of Scotland Coronary Prevention Study

INTRODUCTION

BACKGROUND

Hypertension is a common disorder affecting around one-third of the population in most Western countries. It is a major risk factor for cardiovascular and renal disease, but it is usually asymptomatic and has been referred to as 'the silent killer'. For the past century, hypertension has been the subject of much intensive research and a wealth of high-quality publications. Despite this, however, the aetiology of essential hypertension remains incompletely understood. Indeed, as Churchill said of Russia, hypertension can perhaps still be thought of as 'a riddle wrapped in mystery inside an enigma' (Sir Winston Churchill, 1st October 1939).

Nevertheless, identification and thorough investigation of hypertension do allow a cure for some. Moreover, the benefits of treating hypertension *per se* have been firmly established by major trials. Although a surfeit of anti-hypertensive medications is now available, newer and perhaps better-tolerated therapies are likely to be developed by the pharmaceutical industry in the coming years, and these may help more patients with hypertension to achieve their target blood pressures.

DEFINITIONS

Blood pressure, like many biological variables, has a skewed normal distribution (Fig. 1.1), and there appears to be a continuous linear relationship between blood pressure level and risk. This uni-modal pattern of blood pressure distribution indicates that hypertension is a polygenetic disorder arising as a result of several environmental and/or genetic influences. For these reasons it is impossible to define hypertension, and any definition offered will be purely arbitrary.

For practical purposes, hypertension can be considered as a level of blood pressure that is associated with a significantly increased risk

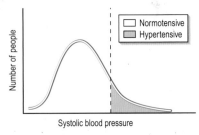

Fig. 1.1 Blood pressure shows a skewed normal distribution within any population.

TABLE 1.1 Categorization of hypertension by severity (JNC 7)

Category	Systolic and diastolic pressure (mmHg)
Normal	< 120 and < 80
Pre-hypertension	120–139 or 80–89
Hypertension stage 1	140–159 or 90–99
Hypertension stage 2	≥ 160 or ≥ 100

(After Chobanian et al 2003, with permission of the National Heart, Lung, and Blood Institute.)

of cardiovascular disease compared with that of the population as a whole, and one at which there is likely to be a benefit treatment. Most specialists would consider a sustained blood pressure of 140/90 mmHg or above as being 'hypertensive' (World Health Organization – International Society of Hypertension definition).

Nevertheless, a significant proportion of hypertension-related disease occurs in those individuals considered to be 'normotensive', because—although the risk is lower in absolute terms—many more people within the population have a blood pressure below 140/90 mmHg than are deemed to be clinically hypertensive. For these reasons the latest Joint National Committee's report on hypertension (JNC 7) refers to a blood pressure over 120/80 mmHg as 'pre-hypertensive' (Table 1.1).[1] Selective lifestyle advice within this population may help to reduce blood pressure levels in general and also the number of individuals who develop sustained hypertension.

ESSENTIAL VERSUS SECONDARY HYPERTENSION

Hypertension may be classified by aetiology into two categories:

● Essential (or primary) hypertension, cause unknown
● Secondary hypertension, where a cause (e.g. renal artery stenosis) has been identified (see *Secondary hypertension*, p. 33).

Essential hypertension is increasingly recognized as a heterogeneous condition, which no doubt reflects the many different contributory factors.

Perhaps the most important clinical distinction is between individuals with isolated systolic hypertension and those with elevated diastolic and/or systolic pressures (Fig. 1.2).

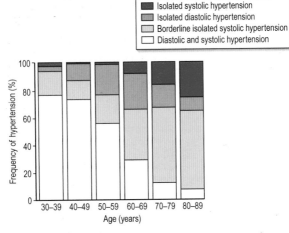

Fig. 1.2 Types of hypertension by age. (From Sagie et al © 1993,[2] Massachusetts Medical Society. All rights reserved.)

- 'Classical' essential hypertension tends to be associated with elevated diastolic and/or systolic pressures and is more common in the under-fifties.
- Isolated systolic hypertension is almost exclusively a disease of older individuals.

Such observations, together with differing underlying pathophysiological causes, reinforce the notion that they are distinct conditions. In a similar manner, much attention has been paid to the distinction between low- and high-renin hypertension. In some respects such a distinction is artificial, but there is increasing evidence that it may provide a guide to the therapeutic response.

ISOLATED SYSTOLIC HYPERTENSION

Isolated systolic hypertension is defined as a raised systolic pressure in conjunction with a normal or even low diastolic pressure (i.e. a widened pulse pressure). Once again, definitions are purely arbitrary but, from a practical point of view, in the UK the British Hypertension Society (BHS) guidelines are used,[3] and in the USA the criteria laid down by JNC 7 (Table 1.2).

Isolated systolic hypertension is a common disorder in Western countries, especially in older individuals. Using the BHS definition, it

TABLE 1.2 Defining isolated systolic hypertension

Organization	Systolic and diastolic pressure (mmHg)
British Hypertension Society	≥ 160 and < 90
Joint National Committee	≥ 140 and < 90
World Health Organization–International Society of Hypertension	≥ 140 and < 90

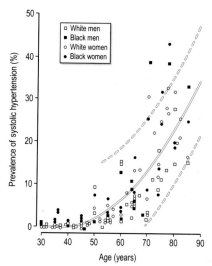

Fig. 1.3 The prevalence of isolated systolic hypertension by age. (From Staessen et al 1990,[4] with permission of Lippincott, Williams and Wilkins.)

is estimated that this condition affects about 25% of those aged over 60 years, but over 50% if the JNC 7 criteria are applied. In contrast, isolated systolic hypertension is uncommon in those younger than 50 years (Fig. 1.3).

MALIGNANT HYPERTENSION

Malignant hypertension, or *accelerated-phase hypertension*, is the term used to describe hypertension associated with retinal haemorrhages and/or papilloedema. Haemolytic anaemia, renal impairment, proteinuria and haematuria may also be present, and the diastolic blood pressure is often but not always greater than 120 mmHg.

Malignant hypertension is usually associated with a rapid rise in arterial pressure, and untreated leads to expeditious end-organ damage including cardiac failure and hypertensive encephalopathy. The incidence of malignant hypertension is about 2 per 100 000 per year, but it is relatively more common in younger adults, males and black people. There is also an increased incidence of secondary hypertension.

WHITE COAT HYPERTENSION

White coat hypertension is used to describe the situation in which an individual's blood pressure is elevated in a clinical situation (e.g. an outpatient clinic) but is 'normal' when assessed outside this setting. It has also been called isolated office hypertension.

REFERENCES

1. Chobanian AV, Bakris GL, Black HR, et al. The seventh report of the Joint National Committee on Prevention, Detection, Evaluation, and Treatment of High Blood Pressure (JNC 7). Bethesda: National Heart, Lung, and Blood Institute; 2003.
2. Sagie A, Larson MG, Levy D. The natural history of borderline isolated systolic hypertension. N Engl J Med 1993; 329: 1912–1917.
3. Williams B, Poulter NR, Brown MJ, et al. Guidelines for management of hypertension: report of the Fourth Working Party of the British Hypertension Society, 2004—BHS IV. J Hum Hypertens 2004; 18: 139–185.
4. Staessen J, Amery A, Fagard R. Isolated systolic hypertension in the elderly. J Hypertens 1990; 8: 393–405.

EPIDEMIOLOGY OF HYPERTENSION

INCIDENCE AND PREVALENCE

Hypertension affects approximately one-third of the population.[1] However, the prevalence of hypertension increases significantly with age, consistent with the age-related rise in blood pressure observed in most populations (Fig. 1.4).[3,4]

The Health Survey for England in 1998 reported the prevalence of hypertension as:

- 16% in those aged 30–40 years
- 36% in those aged 60–69 years
- 50% in those aged 80 years and over.

The overall prevalence of hypertension (140/90 mmHg) was 37%. In the North of England Study, hypertension was identified in 50.3% of primary care patients aged 65–80 years, in whom only:

- 30.0% had achieved adequate blood pressure control (< 150/90 mmHg)

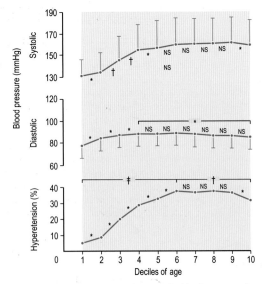

Fig. 1.4 Age and hypertension: trends in systolic blood pressure, diastolic blood pressure and prevalence of hypertension (systolic blood pressure ≥ 160 mmHg or diastolic blood pressure ≥ 95 mmHg) across deciles of age. *, $P < 0.05$; †, $P < 0.01$; ‡, $P < 0.001$. (From Casiglia and Palatini 1998,[2] with permission.)

- 13.5% had attained optimal blood pressure control (< 140/85 mmHg).

These data suggest that the prevalence of hypertension is between 30 and 50% in the over sixty-fives, but that in practice a significantly lower proportion of patients are actually identified, treated, and ultimately attain good blood pressure control.

Essential hypertension accounts for between 90 and 95% of all hypertension, with a variety of secondary causes making up the remainder (see *Secondary hypertension*, p. 33). However, the exact proportions depend on a number of factors, including:

- patient selection
- age
- how hard one looks for a cause.

Malignant hypertension is now very rare in Western societies, although it is relatively more common in younger individuals and in those of African descent.

AGE-RELATED CHANGES IN BLOOD PRESSURE

In almost all societies, systolic blood pressure rises progressively throughout life, whereas diastolic blood pressure rises modestly until the age of 50 years and then falls; thus pulse pressure (systolic minus diastolic pressure) actually increases after middle age (Fig. 1.5).

Until recently, these age-related changes in blood pressure were accepted as an inevitable and benign part of the ageing process. However, we now recognize that such widening of the pulse pressure is associated with a significant increase in cardiovascular morbidity and mortality, and, therefore, can no longer be considered as either physiologically normal or benign. Indeed, pulse pressure increases because of progressive arterial stiffening (arteriosclerosis), a process that appears to be accelerated in certain individuals and in those with established cardiovascular risk factors such as diabetes mellitus.

The age-related changes in blood pressure in modern populations seem to reflect continued exposure to a number of environmental factors, which results in progressive arterial stiffening, rather than any intrinsic physiological process. Evidence supporting this view comes from observations of certain non-urbanized communities in which ageing is not associated with rising blood pressure. For example, in the Kuna island dwellers in the Panamanian Caribbean, blood pressure does not rise through life and hypertension is very uncommon. However, in those islanders who migrate to the urbanized Panama City, the prevalence of hypertension increases to 10.7% and

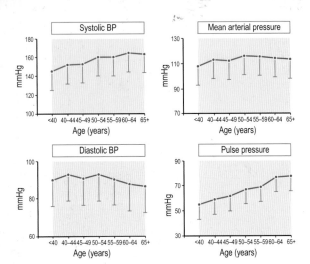

Fig. 1.5 Age and blood pressure: age-related trends in systolic blood pressure, diastolic blood pressure, mean arterial pressure and pulse pressure for each 5-year age group from less than 40 to over 65 years. (From Khattar et al 2001,[5] with permission.)

exceeds 45% in those over 60 years of age, indicating that age-related blood pressure patterns depend on exposure to environmental factors.

REFERENCES

1. Primatesta P, Brookes M, Poulter NR. Improved hypertension management and control: results from the Health Survey for England, 1998. Hypertension 2001; 38(4): 827–832.
2. Casiglia E, Palatini P. Cardiovascular risk factors in the elderly. J Hum Hypertens 1998; 12: 575–581.
3. Franklin SS, Gustin IVW, Wong ND, et al. Hemodynamic patterns of age-related changes in blood pressure: the Framingham Heart Study. Circulation 1997; 96: 308–315.
4. Franklin SS, Jacobs MJ, Wong ND, et al. Predominance of isolated systolic hypertension among middle-aged and elderly US hypertensives: analysis based on National Health and Nutrition Examination Survey (NHANES) III. ▶ Hypertension 2001; 37(3): 869–874.
5. Khattar RS, Swales JD, Dore C. Effect of aging on the prognostic significance of ambulatory systolic, diastolic, and pulse pressure in essential hypertension. Circulation 2001; 104: 783–789.

CONSEQUENCES OF HYPERTENSION

SIGNS AND SYMPTOMS

Essential hypertension is usually asymptomatic and may, therefore, remain undetected for many years. Occasionally headache can occur, particularly when the systolic blood pressure is elevated beyond 200 mmHg, or when blood pressure is rising rapidly, as can occur in malignant hypertension. Therefore, in most cases hypertension is diagnosed on routine blood pressure examination or when a major complication arises. Nevertheless, malignant hypertension is associated with a number of symptoms (Box 1.1) and signs (Table 1.3). Likewise, secondary forms of hypertension may present with a range of non-specific symptoms, such as palpitations, sweating and rashes, due to the underlying disease.

Box 1.1 Symptoms associated with malignant hypertension

Headache
Blurred vision
Chest pain
Breathlessness
Nausea, vomiting
Anxiety, confusion, coma
Seizures

TABLE 1.3 Consequences of malignant hypertension

End organ	Complications
Aorta	Aortic dissection
Brain	Hypertensive encephalopathy Cerebral infarction or haemorrhage
Heart	Cardiac failure Myocardial ischaemia or infarction
Kidney	Renal failure Haematuria
Gastrointestinal	Anorexia, nausea, vomiting, abdominal pain
Placenta	Eclampsia
Other	Micro-angiopathic haemolytic anaemia

Box 1.2 Consequences of hypertension

Cardiac disease
Left ventricular failure
Angina
Myocardial infarction

Cerebrovascular disease
Transient ischaemic attacks
Stroke
Multi-infarct dementia
Hypertensive encephalopathy

Vascular disease
Aortic aneurysm
Occlusive peripheral vascular disease
Arterial dissection

Others
Progressive renal failure
Hypertensive retinopathy

Abnormalities on routine examination in essential hypertension are infrequent, except for retinopathy (see *Clinical assessment of hypertension*, p. 61). However, the consequences of sustained hypertension may become manifest, predominantly in the cardiovascular, cerebrovascular and renovascular systems, as summarized in Box 1.2. Individuals with secondary hypertension may of course present with signs due to the underlying condition.

RISKS OF HYPERTENSION

Hypertension is one of a number of important cardiovascular risk factors that have been identified, including:

- advancing age
- positive family history of premature cardiovascular disease
- diabetes mellitus
- smoking
- hypercholesterolaemia.

Multivariate analysis has been used to determine the particular contribution that blood pressure makes to overall cardiovascular risk,

TABLE 1.4 The relative values of selected risk factors in predicting future stroke

Risk factor	Relative risk
Hypertension	7.0
Diabetes (female)	5.8
Previous transient ischaemic attack	5–13
Left ventricular hypertrophy	4.4
Diabetes (male)	4.1
Atrial fibrillation	3.7
Cardiac disease	3.0

and it appears that hypertension is one of the most significant single, modifiable risk factors. For example, in Western populations hypertension confers up to a seven-fold increase in the risk of stroke (Table 1.4). Furthermore, hypertension is thought to account for:

- one-half of all deaths due to stroke
- up to one-quarter of coronary heart disease deaths.

Consequently there are potentially very substantial opportunities for reducing cardiovascular morbidity and mortality by appropriate identification and management of individuals with raised blood pressure.[1]

The relationship between raised blood pressure and cardiovascular disease risk persists regardless of age (Fig. 1.6). Indeed, the presence of hypertension confers an increased cardiovascular risk at all ages.[2] Likewise, the ingrained views concerning the innocuous nature of isolated systolic hypertension are completely unfounded. Isolated systolic hypertension increases the risk of:

- stroke and coronary heart disease by about 40%
- cardiovascular death by about 50%
- heart failure by about 50%.

For these reasons, hypertension in any form in older individuals cannot be ignored or viewed as part of the normal ageing process.

THE J-SHAPED CURVE

The relationship between blood pressure and risk appears to be linear within the population (Figs 1.7–1.9). However, there has been controversy surrounding the possibility of a lower limit beyond which

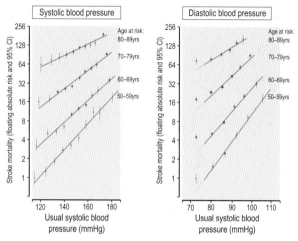

Fig. 1.6 Age, blood pressure, and relative risk of stroke. (From Lewington et al 2002[2], with permission from Elsevier.)

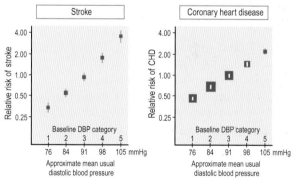

Fig. 1.7 Blood pressure and relative risk of stroke (data from seven prospective observational studies: 843 events) and coronary heart disease (nine prospective observational studies: 4856 events) in five categories defined by baseline diastolic blood pressure. (From McMahon et al 1990[3], with permission from Elsevier.)

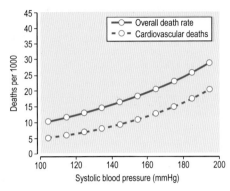

Fig. 1.8 Age-adjusted cardiovascular mortality and systolic blood pressure in the Framingham Study population. (From Port et al 2000[4], with permission from Elsevier.)

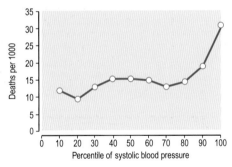

Fig. 1.9 Cardiovascular mortality in the Framingham Study population by systolic blood pressure percentile. (From Port et al 2000[4], with permission from Elsevier.)

lower blood pressures carry an increased risk: the so-called 'J-shaped curve'. Although observational data from the Framingham Study indicate a very clear relationship between rising blood pressure and cardiovascular mortality risk, the lowest blood pressure decile was not associated with lowest overall risk (Fig. 1.9). However, these observational data are heavily confounded by inclusion of individuals who may have had low blood pressure as a manifestation of cardiovascular or other diseases.

In the most recent meta-analysis reported, including data from over one million subjects, there was a continuous relationship between risk and blood pressure down to a systolic pressure of

115 mmHg and a diastolic pressure of 75 mmHg.[2] Moreover, clinical trials of hypertension treatment have failed to demonstrate any lower limit beyond which blood pressure should not be lowered. Therefore the current consensus view is that the relationship between blood pressure and risk is linear.

MALIGNANT HYPERTENSION

Malignant hypertension remains one of the immediate life-threatening complications of blood pressure elevation and is associated with end-organ damage (Table 1.3). Cerebral blood flow is auto-regulated within specific limits, and normally cerebral blood flow remains unchanged between mean arterial pressures of 60 and 120 mmHg. As mean arterial pressure increases, compensatory cerebral vasoconstriction limits cerebral hyperperfusion, but beyond a mean arterial pressure of about 180 mmHg this auto-regulation is overwhelmed and cerebral vasodilatation and oedema ensue.

Previously normotensive individuals can develop signs of encephalopathy at blood pressures as low as 160/100 mmHg, whereas individuals with long-standing hypertension may not do so until the blood pressure rises to 220/110 mmHg or greater. Untreated, the 5-year mortality of malignant hypertension approaches 100%, but this figure is dramatically reduced by pharmacological intervention.

> **Important:** Blood pressure should be reduced gradually in the majority of cases, apart from in true hypertensive emergencies such as encephalopathy, acute left ventricular failure, and aortic dissection.

WHITE COAT HYPERTENSION AND CARDIOVASCULAR RISK

White coat hypertension is often considered to be a benign condition, due in part to the intermittent nature of the blood pressure elevation, frequently in the setting of situational stress or anxiety. However, several lines of evidence suggest that this may not be the case.

- Many early clinical trials that enrolled patients on the basis of serial office recordings probably included patients with white coat hypertension, yet these studies were still able to demonstrate benefit from blood pressure lowering.

- There appears to be a higher prevalence of metabolic abnormalities consistent with the insulin resistance syndrome, possibly mediated by increased sympathetic adrenergic activity in white coat hypertensive individuals.
- Individuals with white coat hypertension or abnormally variable blood pressure appear to be at increased risk of developing sustained hypertension. In a 5-year follow-up study of healthy army personnel, the risk of future hypertension among individuals with transient hypertension at outset was three to six times higher than among normotensive persons.
- Finally, end-organ damage and cardiovascular risk per se in those with white coat hypertension appear to lie between that of normotensive persons and individuals with sustained hypertension.

In view of these observations and the suggestion of increased cardiovascular risk associated with white coat hypertension, anti-hypertensive treatment should be considered appropriate in the majority of cases, especially if there is evidence of end-organ damage. At the very least, individuals with white coat hypertension should be assessed regularly (6–12 monthly) to ensure that they have not developed sustained hypertension.

REFERENCES

1. Franklin SS, Jacobs MJ, Wong ND, et al. Predominance of isolated systolic hypertension among middle-aged and elderly US hypertensives: analysis based on National Health and Nutrition Examination Survey (NHANES) III. Hypertension 2001; 37(3): 869–874
2. Lewington S, Clarke R, Qizilbash N, et al. Age-specific relevance of usual blood pressure to vascular mortality: a meta-analysis of individual data for one million adults in 61 prospective studies. Lancet 2002; 360(9349): 1903–1913.
3. McMahon S, Peto R, Cutler J, et al. Blood pressure, stroke, and coronary heart disease. Part 1, prolonged differences in blood pressure: prospective observational studies corrected for the regression dilution bias. Lancet 1990; 335: 765–774.
4. Port S, Demer L, Jennrich R, et al. Systolic blood pressure and mortality. Lancet 2000; 355: 175–180.

AETIOLOGY OF HYPERTENSION

PATHOPHYSIOLOGY OF ESSENTIAL HYPERTENSION

The exact physiological basis of essential hypertension remains uncertain. However, over the past century our understanding of the mechanisms involved in its pathogenesis has increased substantially. It has also become clear that both genetic and environmental factors contribute to the development of hypertension.

In the very early phase of essential hypertension, cardiac output is thought to be increased, with a relatively normal total peripheral resistance: a so-called 'hyperkinetic' circulation. As hypertension becomes established, cardiac output returns to normal and peripheral vascular resistance is increased. Ultimately cardiac output is lower than in normotensive individuals.

Various structural changes in the resistance vessels (arterioles and arteries less than 300 μm in diameter) from hypertensive patients have been described, including an increase in wall to lumen ratio. This is likely to be due to remodelling, but there is also evidence to suggest hyperplasia of smooth muscle cells in some forms of hypertension. Such changes contribute to the fixed increased peripheral vascular resistance in these patients, but it is unclear whether these changes are primary or secondary. Partial reversal of these changes with anti-hypertensive drugs has been reported, but this appears to be incomplete.

The return of cardiac output to normal is accompanied by resetting of baroreceptor sensitivity to changes in blood pressure, possibly as a consequence of arteriolar medial hyperplasia. Increased systemic vascular resistance and impaired baroreflex sensitivity are both important maladaptive responses that beget further increases in blood pressure.

The pathological hallmark of malignant hypertension is fibrinoid necrosis of the arterioles and hyperplastic arteriolitis of the arterioles and arteries (onion-skinning). There is usually:

- a marked increased in peripheral vascular resistance
- reduction in cardiac output
- activation of the renin–angiotensin system.

In severe cases micro-angiopathic haemolytic anaemia may be present.

THE AUTONOMIC NERVOUS SYSTEM AND HYPERTENSION

Over 100 years ago, Geisbock was among the first to propose that the nervous system may be responsible for the development of essential hypertension. There is evidence that increased sympathetic tone and decreased parasympathetic tone make a substantial contribution to essential hypertension, particularly in younger patients with early, borderline hypertension.

- Total brain, and in particular sub-cortical, turnover of noradrenaline is substantially higher in hypertensive than in normotensive individuals.
- Analysis of heart rate variability has also provided evidence of increased sympathetic and decreased parasympathetic cardiac influences.
- More direct techniques, such as sympathetic microneurography of fibres carried by the common peroneal nerve, also support the view of increased sympathetic neuronal outflow in young hypertensive individuals.

Therefore a large body of evidence, both direct and indirect, suggests that excess sympathetic activity is an important mechanism in essential hypertension, particularly in younger patients.

THE KIDNEY AND HYPERTENSION

Interest in the kidney's involvement in hypertension also dates back to the late 19th century with the isolation and characterization of renin. This was reinforced by the classic experiments in the 1930s by Goldblatt, who demonstrated that temporary renal artery occlusion could lead to the development of permanent hypertension (the 2-kidney 1-clip model).

We now know that the renin–angiotensin system is an important hormonal axis that is responsible for control of:

- renal function
- blood pressure
- fluid and electrolyte balance.

Renin, secreted by the macula densa in the juxta-glomerular apparatus in response to reduced renal blood flow, catalyses the conversion of circulating angiotensinogen to angiotensin I. In turn, this is converted to angiotensin II by angiotensin-converting enzyme (ACE), which is located throughout the body. Angiotensin II is a

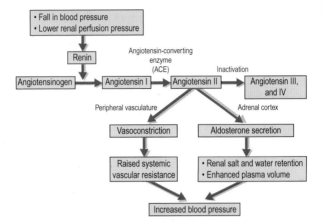

Fig. 1.10 The role of the renin–angiotensin–aldosterone system in the physiological regulation of blood pressure.

potent vasoconstrictor and also stimulates aldosterone release from the adrenal cortex, enhancing renal salt and water retention (Fig. 1.10). All these effects are mediated by the AT_1 receptor.

The renin–angiotensin system, therefore, serves to maintain blood pressure in situations where renal blood flow or blood volume is significantly reduced, and it is comparatively quiescent in healthy, well-hydrated individuals. Interestingly, catecholamines acting via the β adrenoceptor also stimulate renin production, providing a link between the sympathetic nervous system and the kidney.

In a small sub-group of patients with secondary hypertension due to either renal artery stenosis or rare monogenic syndromes (see *Secondary hypertension*, p. 33), the kidney is clearly involved in the origin of hypertension. However, in about 15% of hypertensive individuals with essential hypertension there is significantly and inappropriately elevated plasma renin activity, suggesting that the renin–angiotensin system may play an important role in elevating blood pressure in these individuals. Such patients show a particularly effective blood pressure reduction in response to renin–angiotensin system blockade by:

- β blockers
- ACE inhibitors
- angiotensin receptor antagonists.

Therefore excessive renin–angiotensin system activation appears to contribute to the maintenance of hypertension in a small sub-group of patients, but whether it is more directly involved in the genesis of hypertension more widely continues to be debated.

GENES AND HYPERTENSION

The uni-modal (i.e. continuous) distribution of blood pressure in the population, as well as various family and twin studies, strongly suggest that there is a genetic contribution to the development of hypertension. This view has been reinforced by identification of various, albeit very rare, single gene defects that can lead to hypertension. For example, the autosomal dominant hypertensive syndrome of glucocorticoid-remediable hyperaldosteronism (see *Secondary hypertension*, p. 33) results from a genetic chimerism of the genes encoding 11β-hydroxylase and aldosterone synthase. Further support for the role of genetic abnormalities comes from animal work and the development of genetically inbred animal strains with various forms of hypertension, such as spontaneously hypertensive rats.

Despite the above evidence, it has become apparent that no one single gene is responsible for essential hypertension, which more than likely represents a complex inter-play between many different 'hypertensive genes' and the environment. Nevertheless, there are currently several large studies being conducted in the UK and the USA to try to identify hypertensive loci within the human genome, and then to focus on specific candidate genes. If this approach proves successful, it may ultimately be possible to tailor therapy to the individual based on genotype.

PATHOPHYSIOLOGY OF ISOLATED SYSTOLIC HYPERTENSION

In contrast to classical essential hypertension, isolated systolic hypertension results from stiffening of the large arteries rather than an increase in peripheral vascular resistance or cardiac output. In almost all populations there is an age-related increase in large artery stiffness (Fig. 1.11). This is due to disruption and disorganization of elastic elements (mainly elastin and collagen) within the arterial wall, which result in dilatation and stiffening of the artery: the process of arteriosclerosis (not to be confused with atherosclerosis).

The reason for this 'fatigue fracture' is simple if one considers that by the age of 60 an individual has experienced roughly 2000

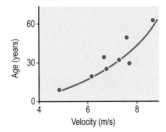

Fig. 1.11 Age and arterial stiffness. Bramwell and Hill were among the first to demonstrate an age-related increase in arterial stiffness (as assessed by the aortic pulse wave velocity). These observations have been subsequently confirmed in much larger populations from both rural and urban communities. (From Bramwell and Hill 1922,[1] with permission from Elsevier.)

million heartbeats, and that with each beat a pulsatile expansion of the large elastic arteries occurs. Nevertheless, certain conditions— such as diabetes, cigarette smoking and hypertension *per se*—are thought to accelerate this phenomenon and thus predispose to systolic hypertension.

Although the above hypothesis is attractive, it would appear that isolated systolic hypertension is not simply the 'burnt out' phase of diastolic hypertension, because fewer than 30% of individuals with isolated systolic hypertension have had diastolic or systolic–diastolic hypertension previously documented.

Important: Isolated systolic hypertension is not a benign condition and is associated with considerable excess cardiovascular morbidity and mortality.

REFERENCE

1. Bramwell JC, Hill AV. Velocity of transmission of the pulse-wave and elasticity of the arteries. Lancet 1922; i: 891–892.

LIFESTYLE FACTORS AND RELATIONSHIP WITH HYPERTENSION

Several lifestyle factors have an influence on blood pressure.

In any individual patient it is important to highlight those lifestyle changes that are most likely to help and to encourage compliance with these, even if the patient is already taking anti-hypertensive medication. In some cases of borderline hypertension, lifestyle changes may produce a reduction in blood pressure sufficient to avoid the need for the introduction of drug therapy.

> **Important:** Although small reductions in blood pressure can be achieved by changing any one lifestyle factor, the best result is obtained if all relevant factors are addressed at the same time.

WEIGHT

Being obese increases the risk of developing hypertension. Moreover, weight and body mass index (BMI) (Table 1.5) correlate with blood pressure even within the normal range.

There are several theories to explain why obesity predisposes to hypertension.

- Sympathetic drive is increased in overweight people, and this may contribute to vasoconstriction and increased renin production by the kidney.
- In addition, obesity is associated with other abnormalities, such as dyslipidaemia and impaired glucose tolerance, which along with hypertension increase overall cardiovascular risk.

TABLE 1.5 Body mass index (BMI; weight (kg)/height (m)^2) and weight category

BMI (kg/m^2)	Category
< 19.0	Underweight
19.0–25.0	Normal weight
25.1–30.0	Overweight
30.1–35.0	Clinically obese
> 35.0	Morbidly obese

Blood pressure falls with weight reduction; therefore weight loss is an obvious early lifestyle intervention in many hypertensive patients. Usually a combination of diet and exercise is recommended. Although it is unlikely that blood pressure reduction of more than a few mmHg will be achieved through weight loss alone, even small amounts of weight loss are beneficial in terms of cardiovascular risk, and in a borderline hypertensive patient it may delay the need for introduction of drug therapy.

SALT INTAKE

The relationship between dietary salt intake and blood pressure has been the subject of much debate over the past 50 years. However, salt intake would appear to influence blood pressure in at least some patients.

The INTERSALT study looked at the relationship between salt intake and blood pressure in 10 079 individuals.[1] Using 24-hour urinary sodium excretion as a marker of salt intake, the study found a significant positive relationship between sodium excretion and systolic blood pressure (Fig. 1.12). The association was stronger in older people, whom we know from other studies tend to have a higher aldosterone to renin ratio.

Several randomized trials have shown that reduction of dietary salt intake is successful in reducing blood pressure. Again, the amount of blood pressure reduction achievable varies between patients, with some tending to be more salt-sensitive than others. Work in rats has identified the presence of quantitative trait loci for

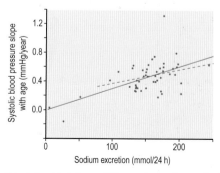

Fig. 1.12 The relationship between 24-hour urinary salt excretion (as a measure of salt intake) and systolic blood pressure in the INTERSALT study. (From Rose and Stamler 1989,[1] with permission.)

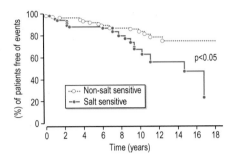

Fig. 1.13 Prognosis based on salt sensitivity. (From Morimoto et al 1997,[2] with permission from Elsevier.)

salt sensitivity of blood pressure on several chromosomes; therefore it is likely that there is also genetic variability in human salt sensitivity. Salt-sensitive patients—defined as having at least 10 mmHg difference in systolic blood pressure between high- and low-salt diets—have a poorer prognosis than non-salt-sensitive patients (Fig. 1.13).

Reductions in blood pressure with salt restriction are greater in hypertensive than in normotensive people, per 100-mmol decrease in daily sodium intake:

- approximately 6 mmHg systolic and 2 mmHg diastolic in hypertensive individuals
- 1 mmHg systolic in normotensive individuals.

Salt restriction is a useful adjunct to pharmacological treatment of hypertension, complementing the actions of thiazide diuretics and combination regimens. In a borderline hypertensive patient, careful salt restriction may obviate the need for drug therapy, at least temporarily. However, it is unlikely that blood pressure will fall more than a few mmHg on a salt restriction diet, and some patients will find that the degree of salt restriction necessary to achieve this makes their diet unpalatable. Nonetheless, it is true that salt intake is habit-forming, and that after a deliberate reduction in salt intake it takes only a few weeks for the taste buds to readjust and for one to stop noticing the loss of flavour.

It seems sensible to recommend to hypertensive patients that they should avoid adding extra salt to their food at the table and preferably also during cooking. In particular they should avoid regular intake of crisps, salted nuts, and processed or pre-prepared foods including soups and 'ready meals', which tend to have a high salt content. The use of alternative flavourings in cooking, such as herbs and pepper, may improve taste while avoiding extra salt intake. There are also commercially available salt alternatives containing potassium in place of sodium. These preparations taste similar to regular salt but do not increase the blood pressure.

ALCOHOL

There is a positive linear relationship between alcohol consumption and blood pressure in both men and women. In addition to the changes in blood pressure associated with chronic alcohol intake, acute alcohol intake also raises blood pressure. Aside from total alcohol intake, binge drinking patterns of intake are thought to increase cardiovascular risk.

The relationship between alcohol intake and total cardiovascular risk is complicated, and it was originally thought to be depicted by a so-called 'J-shaped curve' with a higher risk in heavier drinkers and non-drinkers than in moderate alcohol drinkers. It is not clear whether the increased cardiovascular risk in non-drinkers is a genuine finding or whether results are confounded by the inclusion of people with other health problems in the non-drinking group. More recent studies have failed to demonstrate such a relationship, although it is clear that risk increases with increasing alcohol intake beyond a moderate intake.

Reduction of alcohol intake in hypertensive patients leads to a reduction in blood pressure of up to 5–8 mmHg systolic and 2–3 mmHg diastolic. Although these changes may seem small, they are about equivalent to the effect of one anti-hypertensive agent. Also, a reduction in alcohol intake may help patients to achieve a degree of weight loss. In general it is recommended that hypertensive patients should preferably moderate their alcohol intake to less than 2 units/day.

EXERCISE

Although the acute effects of exercise are to raise blood pressure, in the longer term regular moderate exercise reduces blood pressure by as much as 8 mmHg systolic and 4 mmHg diastolic, and it may also regress left ventricular hypertrophy. Maximal benefit is seen with moderate exercise in patients who were previously sedentary. Blood pressure-lowering effects of exercise are over and above any consequent reduction in BMI, although exercise is more effective if also combined with weight reduction.

The optimal frequency and duration of exercise necessary to achieve these benefits are not known. However, it appears that moderate exercise of 45–60 minutes' duration three or four times per week is as good as more vigorous or daily exercise. Dynamic exercise such as walking, swimming and cycling is preferable to resistance types of exercise such as weightlifting.

REFERENCES

1. Rose G, Stamler J. The INTERSALT study: background, methods and main results. INTERSALT Co-operative Research Group. J Hum Hypertens 1989; 3(5): 283–288.
2. Morimoto A, Uzu T, Fujii T, et al. Sodium sensitivity and cardiovascular events in patients with essential hypertension. Lancet 1997; 350: 1734–1737.

SECONDARY HYPERTENSION

Secondary hypertension is the term used to describe the situation where there is an underlying cause for the elevation in blood pressure. It accounts for around 5–10% of cases of hypertension.

Secondary hypertension is more common in younger patients and in patients who are resistant to anti-hypertensive therapy. The most common cause of secondary hypertension is renal disease, which accounts for around 50% of all cases.

> **Important:** Unlike essential hypertension, it may be possible to cure secondary hypertension by treatment of the underlying cause, therefore it is vital that it is considered in every hypertensive patient.

RENAL PARENCHYMAL DISEASE

Almost all forms of renal parenchymal disease may lead to hypertension. Some of the most common causes are:

- the glomerulonephritides (Fig. 1.14)
- diabetic nephropathy
- chronic pyelonephritis (Fig. 1.15)
- analgesic nephropathy
- adult polycystic kidney disease (Fig. 1.16).

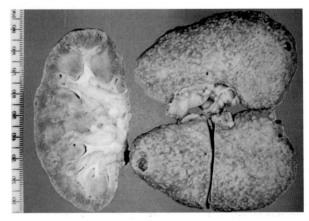

Fig. 1.14 Glomerulonephritis.

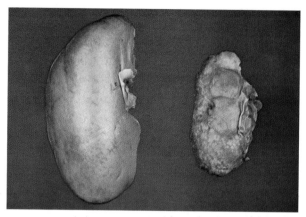

Fig. 1.15 Chronic pyelonephritis. Note the considerable difference in size between the two kidneys. The affected kidney is small and misshapen due to chronic pyelonephritis.

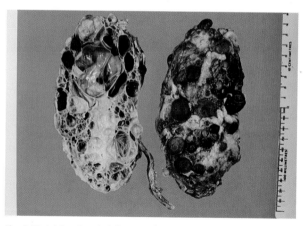

Fig. 1.16 Adult polycystic kidney disease.

Chronic renal failure of any cause is also associated with hypertension.

In some cases pre-existing renal disease will be apparent, otherwise the diagnosis can be reached by history (e.g. use of analgesics or positive family history of polycystic kidney disease), examination (e.g. palpable enlarged kidneys in polycystic disease), and appropriate investigations. Investigations may include:

- serum creatinine and glucose measurement
- urinalysis
- urinary microalbuminuria or proteinuria
- renal ultrasound.

In some cases renal biopsy may be necessary to establish the diagnosis. Treatment of the underlying renal disease will in many cases improve the hypertension; however, it will often be necessary to control the blood pressure with one or more anti-hypertensive agents. Likewise, adequate blood pressure control will reduce the rate of decline of glomerular filtration rate and delay the onset of end-stage renal failure.

RENAL ARTERY STENOSIS

Renal artery stenosis (renovascular disease) occurs in two distinct forms.

- Young people tend to be affected by fibromuscular dysplasia.
- Older people tend to have an atherosclerotic narrowing of the renal arteries.

In both forms the narrowing of the renal arteries restricts blood flow to the kidney, and this causes a reflex increase in renin release from the juxta-glomerular apparatus in the distal tubule of the nephron. Renin acts on angiotensinogen produced by the liver, converting it to angiotensin I. This angiotensin I is then converted to angiotensin II by angiotensin-converting enzyme (ACE) present in the lungs and other tissues. Angiotensin II is a potent vasoconstrictor, increasing peripheral vascular resistance.

Angiotensin II also stimulates aldosterone release from the adrenal cortex, which acts via the mineralocorticoid receptor to increase sodium and water retention (see Fig. 1.10, p. 24). Thus the increased renin leads to hypertension. If the narrowing of the renal arteries is severe and bilateral, there may also be a decline in renal function due to a reduction in glomerular filtration rate. In unilateral renal artery stenosis, the affected kidney may actually be relatively protected from the effects of the systemic hypertension due to the narrowing of the renal artery. In such a case it is the contralateral kidney that will suffer the long-term histological changes associated with hypertension.

> ⚠ **Renal bruits may be present when auscultating over the abdomen or the back. However, this clinical sign is unreliable: the diagnosis must be confirmed by further imaging.**

Renal artery stenosis may be suspected in patients who are either very young or are older with other known atherosclerotic disease. Possible imaging modalities include:

- magnetic resonance angiography
- conventional angiography
- the radioisotope MAG3 scan with captopril challenge.

The last of these gives useful information about the relative function of the two kidneys. Renal ultrasound is not diagnostic, but it may show a discrepancy in the relative size of the kidneys if there is unilateral renal artery stenosis. Doppler ultrasound can be used to measure flow in the renal arteries (Fig. 1.17).

Fibromuscular dysplasia and atherosclerotic renal artery stenosis can be differentiated from each other on angiography.

- Fibromuscular dysplasia may show up as a corkscrew appearance of the renal artery on angiography (Fig. 1.18).
- Atherosclerotic renal artery stenosis usually appears as one or more distinct tight stenoses, often in the proximal renal artery and often accompanied by atherosclerotic disease of the aorta (Fig. 1.19).

Fibromuscular dysplasia responds well to radiological intervention with balloon angioplasty and stenting. Often the blood pressure may return to normal by a few days after the procedure. Patients should be monitored for recurrence of the stenosis, which is usually identified by a rise in the blood pressure.

In contrast, the blood pressure in atherosclerotic renal artery stenosis responds less well to angioplasty and stenting, and the procedure is considerably more risky in older patients with atherosclerotic arteries. The current view is that if blood pressure control can be achieved on medical therapy and there is no compromise of renal function due to the stenosis, anti-hypertensive drug therapy is preferred for these patients. If the blood pressure is poorly controlled on drug therapy, or if there is a severe restriction to

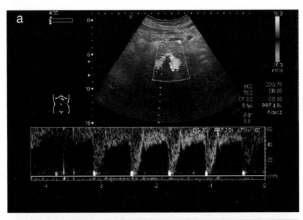

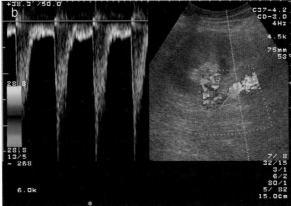

Fig. 1.17 Doppler ultrasound used to measure flow in the renal arteries: (**a**) normal flow and (**b**) renal artery stenosis.

blood flow in the kidney, it may be beneficial to attempt angioplasty and stenting.

In renal artery stenosis, ACE inhibitors may worsen the renal function, especially if the condition is bilateral; however, along with the angiotensin receptor antagonists, they may have a useful role in controlling the blood pressure in such patients, but only under specialist supervision.

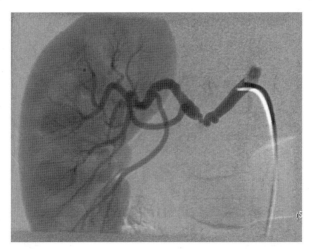

Fig. 1.18 Angiography of the renal artery, showing typical corkscrew appearance of fibromuscular dysplasia.

> **Important:** Therapy with either an ACE inhibitor or an angiotensin receptor antagonist should be started by a specialist, with careful monitoring of renal function 7–10 days after starting therapy and again after any dose increase. If the patient's renal function does not deteriorate significantly, the therapy may be continued.

Other drugs may be required in combination to successfully control the blood pressure in these patients.

PRIMARY HYPERALDOSTERONISM

Primary hyperaldosteronism is due to excessive secretion of the mineralocorticoid hormone aldosterone from the zona glomerulosa of the adrenal gland. There are two main causes of the condition.

- Over-secretion of aldosterone by bilaterally hyperplasic adrenal glands, which is known as bilateral adrenal hyperplasia.
- An adrenal adenoma producing aldosterone, a condition that is usually unilateral and also known as Conn's syndrome.

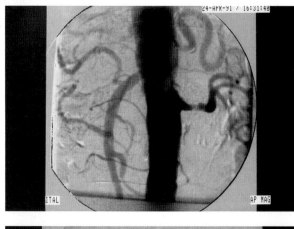

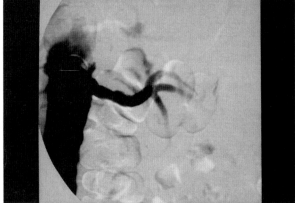

Fig. 1.19 Angiography of the renal artery: (**a**) atherosclerotic renal artery stenosis; (**b**) normal flow is restored following balloon angioplasty of the stricture.

The Conn's adenoma is characteristically canary yellow in appearance on histological section (Fig. 1.20) and is benign. Very rarely, adrenal carcinoma may produce excessive aldosterone secretion; however, adrenal carcinomas are usually non-functional.

Primary hyperaldosteronism usually presents as hypertension that is resistant to therapy. It may also be associated with characteristic electrolyte abnormalities, including:

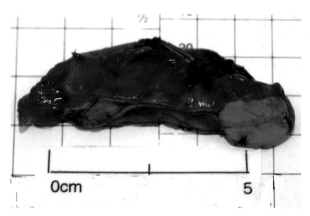

Fig. 1.20 Conn's adenoma in a resected adrenal gland specimen showing the characteristic canary yellow appearance of the cut surface.

- hypokalaemia
- hypernatraemia
- elevated bicarbonate levels.

However, such electrolyte abnormalities are often not present. Most patients are asymptomatic unless they have profound hypokalaemia that may lead to muscle cramps and weakness. Further investigations will detect an elevated plasma aldosterone level associated with a suppressed renin level.

Imaging of the adrenal glands by computerized tomography (CT) or magnetic resonance imaging (MRI) may reveal either a unilateral Conn's adenoma (Fig. 1.21) or bilateral adrenal hyperplasia (Fig. 1.22). Sometimes it can be difficult to determine the probable diagnosis from the scan appearances, particularly in the case of a small adenoma or the presence of multiple nodules in the adrenal glands. In addition, around 5% of the general population will have an abnormal mass in one of their adrenal glands on imaging, the so-called 'adrenal incidentaloma', which may be of no clinical or functional significance. Therefore the presumptive diagnosis should be confirmed by selective adrenal venous sampling (Fig. 1.23) before any definitive diagnosis is made.

In this diagnostic procedure, a venous catheter is inserted into the femoral vein and fed upwards into the inferior vena cava. The catheter is manipulated into the renal and adrenal veins under radiological guidance, and samples of venous blood are collected from:

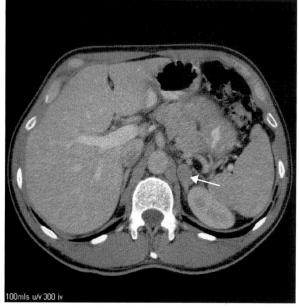

Fig. 1.21 An MRI scan of the abdomen, showing a Conn's adenoma (arrow).

- the adrenal veins
- the renal veins
- the inferior vena cava above the renal veins
- the inferior vena cava below the renal veins.

An arterial blood sample is also obtained via arterial puncture. The blood samples are analysed for their aldosterone and cortisol levels. The cortisol levels help to establish that the catheter was indeed correctly placed in the adrenal veins at the time of the adrenal vein sample collection. The ratio of aldosterone to cortisol in each of the samples is calculated and the values from the various sampling sites compared.

Conn's adenoma can be differentiated from bilateral adrenal hyperplasia as follows.

- In the case of a Conn's adenoma, the aldosterone to cortisol ratio should be markedly higher on the side of the lesion, with suppression of the aldosterone secretion from the other adrenal gland.

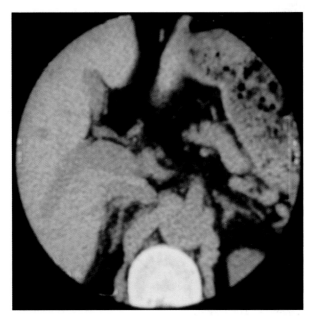

Fig. 1.22 A CT scan of the abdomen, showing bilateral adrenal hyperplasia.

- In the case of bilateral adrenal hyperplasia, the aldosterone to cortisol ratio in adrenal vein blood will be elevated on both sides, and there will be no significant difference between the levels on the two sides.

Some anti-hypertensive therapies may make interpretation of this investigation difficult.

If bilateral adrenal hyperplasia is the diagnosis, surgery is not helpful and the optimal management is medical. The aldosterone antagonist spironolactone is the first-choice agent to control the blood pressure. Doses of around 1 mg/kg daily are usually required to achieve blood pressure control. However, a dose-related side effect of spironolactone is gynaecomastia, and if this becomes troublesome the dose should either be reduced or the alternative potassium-sparing diuretic amiloride may be given instead. A new, more specific aldosterone antagonist, eplerenone, which is thought to cause less gynaecomastia, may soon be available. The above agents may be combined with other anti-hypertensive agents to bring the blood pressure down to target.

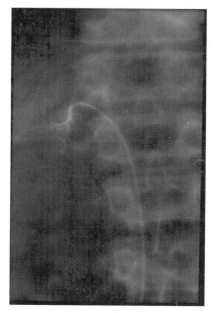

Fig. 1.23 Selective adrenal venous sampling. A catheter is inserted via the femoral vein and fed upwards under radiological guidance. Blood samples are collected from the adrenal and renal veins and inferior vena cava for analysis of aldosterone and cortisol levels.

In the case of a diagnosis of unilateral Conn's adenoma, the options for management are either medical or surgical. Again, spironolactone or amiloride may be used alone or in combination with other anti-hypertensive agents to achieve blood pressure control. However, a more definitive solution to the problem may be gained by removing the adenoma. In practice this requires unilateral adrenalectomy, because it would be very difficult to remove the adenoma in isolation. Nowadays this procedure can often be performed laparoscopically, reducing the length of hospital stay and recovery time following the surgery. However, in some cases an open surgical procedure will be required.

Following removal of the adenoma, the patient may not require any further anti-hypertensive therapy for blood pressure control. However, in cases in which the hypertension has been more long-standing, changes in the vasculature may already have occurred, leading to sustained hypertension and resulting in the patient still needing some anti-hypertensive therapy, although usually fewer drugs will be required than prior to removal of the adenoma. After removal of the adenoma it is no longer necessary to include spironolactone in the anti-hypertensive regimen, and the choice of agent will depend on the patient's age and individual preferences.

The risks and benefits of surgical management of Conn's syndrome should be discussed with the patient, and a decision made jointly as to how to proceed. If there is a high operative risk due to other health problems, or if the patient wishes to avoid surgery for any other reason, it is possible to continue medical management with a combination of spironolactone or amiloride and other anti-hypertensive agents in the long term.

PHAEOCHROMOCYTOMA

Phaeochromocytoma (Fig. 1.24) is a tumour derived of chromaffin cells secreting catecholamines; it is also a rare cause of hypertension, with a prevalence of less than 0.3% in the hypertensive population. The tumour is most commonly located unilaterally in the adrenal medulla, but around 10% are bilateral and 10% are extra-adrenal (although usually intra-abdominal). Phaeochromocytomas may secrete a number of other biologically active substances, including:

- calcitonin
- vasoactive intestinal peptide
- somatostatin
- encephalins
- endorphins
- serotonin
- atrial natriuretic peptide.

Most phaeochromocytomas are benign; however, up to 10% may be malignant, and it is often difficult to differentiate histologically between malignant and benign phaeochromocytomas (although evidence of distant metastases indicates malignancy). There is a higher incidence of malignancy in phaeochromocytomas that are extra-adrenal in location. The genetic basis of phaeochromocytoma is not yet fully understood. In most cases there is no family history; however, phaeochromocytoma is a recognized feature of some inherited syndromes (see Table 1.6).

The clinical features of phaeochromocytoma are highly variable, depending on the pattern of secretion of adrenaline, noradrenaline, and other vasoactive substances. Some patients have very few symptoms and may remain undiagnosed for several years, whereas

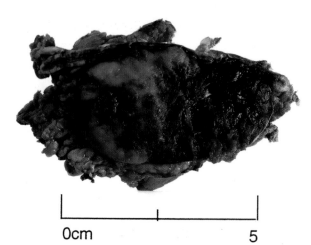

Fig. 1.24 Phaeochromocytoma in a resected adrenal gland specimen. Areas of haemorrhage and necrosis are often seen within the tumour.

TABLE 1.6 Inherited syndromes that may include phaeochromocytoma as a feature	
Inherited syndrome	*Features*
Multiple endocrine neoplasia type IIa	Medullary carcinoma of the thyroid Hyperparathyroidism Phaeochromocytoma
Multiple endocrine neoplasia type IIb	Medullary carcinoma of the thyroid Ganglioneuromatosis Hypertrophy of the corneal nerves Phaeochromocytoma
von Hippel–Lindau disease	Retinal haemangiomas Cerebellar haemangioblastomas Phaeochromocytoma
Neurofibromatosis	Multiple neurofibromas Phaeochromocytoma (rarely)

others have marked episodic symptoms. Most patients have some degree of hypertension, although in some this may be present only episodically. The most common symptoms of phaeochromocytoma are listed in Box 1.3.

Acute hypertensive crises may occur due to surges of release of catecholamines triggered by mechanical compression of the tumour, for example following particular movements, micturition or

---

Box 1.3 Symptoms of phaeochromocytoma

Headache
Sweating attacks accompanied by pallor
Fast palpitations
Feelings of anxiety
Chest pain
Abdominal pain
Nausea
Vomiting
Weight loss
Breathlessness
Blurred vision
Dizziness
Faints
Seizures

---

exercise, or by sudden haemorrhage into the tumour, which is highly vascular.

Hypertensive crises may be complicated by:

- cerebral haemorrhage or infarction
- myocardial infarction
- acute pulmonary oedema
- cardiac arrhythmias including ventricular fibrillation.

Diagnosis of phaeochromocytoma involves confirmation of increased catecholamine secretion, followed by localization of the tumour. The best screening test is a 24-hour urine collection for vanillylmandelic acid or urinary metanephrine and normetanephrine. At least three 24-hour collections should be made before phaeochromocytoma is excluded in patients who have the clinical features of phaeochromocytoma. Plasma adrenaline and noradrenaline levels can be measured to confirm the diagnosis, although these may not be elevated if there is only intermittent excessive secretion of catecholamines, and these may also be affected by factors such as fear of venepuncture.

If there is doubt about the diagnosis, a clonidine suppression test may be helpful. This test involves the administration of the drug clonidine with baseline and repeated measurements of blood pressure and plasma catecholamines. Phaeochromocytoma and essential hypertension without phaeochromocytoma can be differentiated as follows.

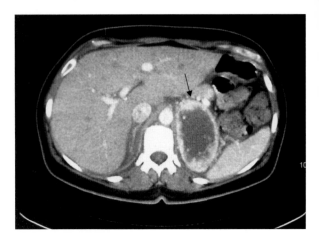

Fig. 1.25 An MRI scan of the abdomen, showing an adrenal phaeochromocytoma (arrow).

- In phaeochromocytoma, the blood pressure will fall but the plasma catecholamines will remain constant.
- In cases of essential hypertension without phaeochromocytoma, both the blood pressure and the plasma catecholamines will fall in response to clonidine.

Once the biochemical diagnosis of phaeochromocytoma has been made, imaging is used to identify the site of the tumour. Because more than 90% of phaeochromocytomas are located in the adrenal glands, CT or MRI of the abdomen is the investigation of choice (Fig. 1.25). If no tumour is seen in the abdomen, it is necessary to perform further imaging to locate the tumour.

If there are specific clues as to the probable anatomical location of the tumour, further CT or MRI techniques may be used, otherwise ^{131}I-metaiodobenzylguanidine (MIBG) scintigraphy scanning is employed (Fig. 1.26). In this technique, labelled MIBG is administered intravenously. The isotope accumulates in phaeochromocytoma tissue as well as in other sites of normal physiological uptake. Images are taken using a gamma camera to identify any abnormal areas of uptake. This technique will also demonstrate the presence of any metastases elsewhere.

More recently, positron emission tomography scanning techniques have been used to localize phaeochromocytomas; however, at present these are expensive and not widely available. Venous catheterization

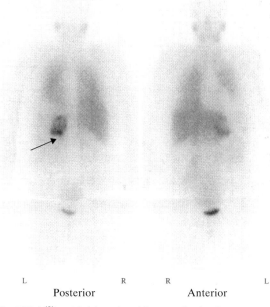

Fig. 1.26 A ^{131}I-metaiodobenzylguanidine scan showing the presence of abnormal isotope uptake in the region of an adrenal phaeochromocytoma (arrow).

of the vena cava via the femoral vein, with collection of blood samples from various levels of the vena cava for analysis for catecholamine levels, is occasionally used where other techniques have failed to localize the tumour.

As soon as the diagnosis of phaeochromocytoma has been made, the patient should be started on specific medication to block the effects of the excess catecholamines. The first agent to be started should be phenoxybenzamine, an irreversible α-adrenoceptor antagonist. A β blocker may then be added to control the resulting tachycardia. The doses of these medications should be escalated until the blood pressure and symptoms are controlled. The medications should be given for around 6 weeks before surgical removal of the tumour is attempted, to allow time for the body to adjust to the lack of catecholamines. In the few days immediately prior to surgery, the patient should be admitted to hospital and the dose of the α blocker gradually increased until postural hypotension is present, usually aiming for a systolic blood pressure drop on standing of at least 20 mmHg. This ensures that the patient is as fluid-replete as possible prior to surgical removal of the tumour.

Surgery can be performed either laparoscopically or as an open procedure. The medication is stopped on the morning of the surgery, and there is usually no need for any anti-hypertensive therapy in the immediate post-operative period. Providing the above pre-operative procedure has been followed, it is unlikely that there will be any major problems with blood pressure control during the operation. However, if there are intra-operative blood pressure changes, the intravenous α blocker phentolamine may be used to control hypertension. Due to the pre-operative α blockade, patients would be relatively insensitive to adrenaline or noradrenaline as pressors; therefore intra-operative hypotension should be treated with intravenous fluids and, if necessary, an intravenous infusion of angiotensin II.

Whether or not a patient will require continuing anti-hypertensive therapy following removal of phaeochromocytoma depends on two factors:

● the duration of presence of the phaeochromocytoma
● the extent of permanent vascular changes that have occurred over time as a result of the excessive release of catecholamines.

Patients should be followed up in the long term on at least an annual basis to screen for recurrence or the development of a second phaeochromocytoma. Patients are screened by measuring 24-hour urine vanillylmandelic acid or plasma catecholamines and blood pressure. All patients who have had a phaeochromocytoma should have the following investigations:

● careful family history to check for the presence of one of the familial syndromes
● calcitonin levels to screen for medullary carcinoma of the thyroid
● parathyroid hormone measurement
● ophthalmological examination to look for features of von Hippel–Lindau disease.

Genetic tests are available to confirm the diagnosis in some cases. Appropriate screening of family members and genetic counselling should be provided if necessary.

Malignant phaeochromocytoma, which accounts for less than 10% of cases, is treated by a combination of surgery, therapeutic ^{131}I-MIBG and chemotherapy.

Pseudophaeochromocytoma is a diagnosis that should be considered in patients presenting with paroxysmal hypertension and many of the typical symptoms of phaeochromocytoma, but in whom catecholamine levels are relatively normal and no phaeochromocytoma tumour is found. This condition is thought to be related to emotional trauma and has also been reported in association with certain drug therapies.

AORTIC COARCTATION

Aortic coarctation is a congenital narrowing of the aorta, most commonly occurring just distal to the origin of the left subclavian artery. The degree of narrowing may vary from a distinct tight band to a more extensive lesion involving a segment of aorta. Coarctation results in hypertension in the upper body, the mechanism of which is thought to be impaired renal artery perfusion resulting in activation of the renin–angiotensin–aldosterone system.

The prevalence of coarctation is around 1 in 10 000, and it is twice as common in males than in females. It is usually diagnosed in childhood, when it presents with hypertension or cardiac failure, although a significant proportion of cases may not present until adolescence or early adulthood. Occasionally it may present as malignant hypertension. Associated abnormalities include a bicuspid aortic valve (in 50% of cases) and cerebral aneurysms. Coarctation is also a recognized feature of Turner's syndrome.

On clinical examination, signs of coarctation include:

- hypertension in the arm, with a systolic blood pressure difference of at least 10 mmHg between the arms and the legs
- diminished or delayed femoral pulses (radio-femoral delay)
- a systolic murmur heard over the back, which may be continuous if the coarctation is severe
- a forceful apex beat, due to left ventricular hypertrophy.

There may also be an associated aortic systolic murmur if there is a bicuspid aortic valve.

Plasma renin activity is usually elevated in cases of coarctation of the aorta. The results of other investigations are as follows.

- Electrocardiography typically shows left ventricular hypertrophy.
- Chest X-ray may show a dilated ascending aorta and rib notching caused by collateral vessels eroding the ribs (Fig. 1.27).
- Echocardiography shows left ventricular hypertrophy and may show the coarctation itself or the presence of a bicuspid aortic valve.

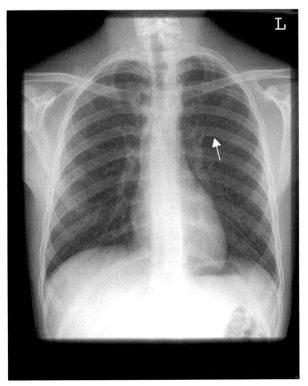

Fig. 1.27 Chest radiograph showing dilated ascending aorta and rib notching due to aortic coarctation.

The diagnosis, site and extent of the lesion are confirmed by imaging of the aorta using CT, MRI or conventional aortography (Fig. 1.28).

The definitive treatment for aortic coarctation is surgical correction, which has the best outcome if performed in childhood between the ages of 1 and 7 years. If correction is not performed until after the age of 7 years, patients are more likely to have long-term hypertension. Even with correction, around 20% of patients will remain hypertensive, probably due to permanent structural and neurohormonal changes in the cardiovascular system. Recurrence of the stenosis occurs in up to 10% of cases operated in childhood. Balloon angioplasty has been used successfully in some cases of recurrence; however, other cases may require repeat surgery.

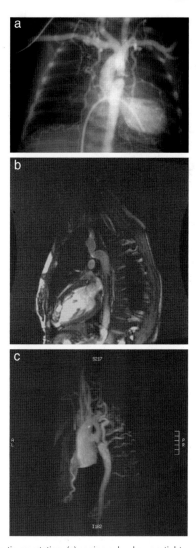

Fig. 1.28 Aortic coarctation: (**a**) angiography shows a tight constriction of the lumen of the descending aorta; (**b**) magnetic resonance angiogram, sagittal view, showing coarctation of the aorta; (**c**) magnetic resonance angiogram showing tight constriction of the descending aorta and prominent collateral vessels.

CUSHING'S SYNDROME

Cushing's syndrome (Fig. 1.29) is a state of glucocorticoid excess that results in hypertension in addition to other typical features listed in Box 1.4.

Non-iatrogenic Cushing's syndrome is most commonly due to a pituitary adenoma secreting excessive amounts of adrenocorticotrophic hormone (ACTH), which stimulates the adrenal gland to produce excessive amounts of cortisol. This is the classical Cushing's disease, which was originally described in 1912 by the American neurosurgeon Harvey Cushing (1869–1939). Cushing's syndrome may also be caused by ectopic ACTH secretion, for example from small-cell lung carcinoma.

The most common cause of Cushing's syndrome is, however, iatrogenic, due to therapy with synthetic glucocorticoids such as prednisolone. Also, ACTH given as a therapy may cause Cushing's syndrome. Other causes include:

● adrenal adenomas
● adrenal hyperplasia
● adrenal carcinomas producing glucocorticoids.

The diagnosis of Cushing's syndrome is usually apparent from the drug history, clinical examination findings, and the presence of impaired glucose tolerance and hypertension; however, in some cases it may not be obvious. If drug therapy as a cause has been excluded,

---

Box 1.4 Features of Cushing's syndrome

Moon face
Truncal obesity
Buffalo hump
Purple abdominal striae
Thin skin
Easy bruising
Hirsutism
Myopathy
Glucose intolerance
Cataracts
Osteoporosis
Menstrual irregularity
Impotence
Depression
Poor wound healing

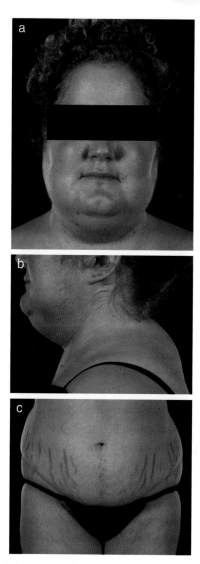

Fig. 1.29 Typical appearance of Cushing's syndrome: (**a**) moon face; (**b**) buffalo hump and hirsutism; (**c**) obesity and abdominal striae.

the diagnosis is made by measuring 24-hour urinary free cortisol levels. Plasma cortisol levels may also be elevated and there is typically loss of diurnal variation. The diagnosis can be confirmed by performing a low-dose dexamethasone suppression test, which will demonstrate a lack of suppression of cortisol secretion.

To differentiate between the various forms of Cushing's syndrome, a high-dose dexamethasone suppression test and ACTH measurements may be performed.

- In true Cushing's disease (due to pituitary adenoma), plasma ACTH will be high or high normal, and cortisol secretion will be suppressed by the high-dose dexamethasone suppression test.
- In cases of ectopic ACTH production, plasma ACTH is usually very high and plasma cortisol will not suppress following dexamethasone.
- If the Cushing's syndrome is due to an adrenal adenoma, plasma ACTH concentration is usually normal, and there is little or no suppression of plasma cortisol levels following dexamethasone.
- In adrenal carcinoma, plasma ACTH levels are usually low and cortisol levels do not suppress following dexamethasone.

In cases of ectopic ACTH secretion, ACTH stimulation tests will show normal cortisol responses. There will be no response in adrenal carcinoma cases.

Localization of tumours is performed using CT or MRI scanning. Selective venous sampling may also be helpful in some cases.

Treatment depends on the underlying cause but usually involves surgical excision of any tumour. Pituitary irradiation may reduce recurrence following removal of a pituitary adenoma. Adrenal carcinoma has a poor prognosis, but chemotherapy may be given as an adjunct to surgery. Unilateral adrenal adenoma responds well to unilateral adrenalectomy, which may be performed laparoscopically or by open procedure. Treatment of ectopic ACTH production involves treatment of the underlying tumour. Medical therapies of some benefit in Cushing's syndrome include:

- the β-hydroxylase inhibitor metyrapone
- the serotonin antagonist cyproheptadine
- the dopamine agonists bromocriptine and lisuride
- the antifungal agent ketoconazole, which reduces steroid synthesis
- mitotane, which destroys the zona reticularis and fasciculata of the adrenal glands.

The hypertension associated with Cushing's syndrome will usually resolve following definitive treatment of the underlying disorder or withdrawal of the causative drug therapy. If the patient is dependent on taking glucocorticoids for control of a coexisting condition and it is not possible to withdraw the steroids, the hypertension is managed using a combination of anti-hypertensive agents.

DRUG-INDUCED HYPERTENSION

THE ORAL CONTRACEPTIVE PILL

One of the most commonly prescribed agents causing hypertension is the combined oral contraceptive pill, which contains a combination of an oestrogen (such as oestradiol) and a progesterone. In most women taking the combined oral contraceptive pill, a small rise in blood pressure occurs, usually of the degree of around a 5-mmHg increase in systolic blood pressure, which is of little significance unless they already have borderline essential hypertension. However, some women seem particularly sensitive to the combined oral contraceptive pill and may have more dramatic increases in blood pressure. If this occurs, the best approach is to stop the combined oral contraceptive pill for a few months and reassess the blood pressure. Often the progesterone-only pill may be a suitable alternative for these women. However, a very small proportion of women have blood pressure increases on the progesterone-only pill, in which case alternative methods of contraception must be advised.

The combined oral contraceptive pill should not be prescribed to women who are already hypertensive, and regular blood pressure checks are advised for women who choose this form of contraception.

OTHER DRUGS

Other drugs that may cause hypertension include:

- steroids (see p. 55)
- non-steroidal anti-inflammatory drugs
- immunosuppressives, such as ciclosporin and tacrolimus
- sympathomimetics, such as ephedrine
- anabolic steroids
- erythropoietin
- monoamine oxidase inhibitors.

Cocaine and amphetamines may induce acute hypertension. Also, substances contained in common foods and drinks, including caffeine and liquorice, may cause hypertension. Liquorice contains a substance called glycyrrhetinic acid, which results in sodium retention, potassium loss, and a rise in blood pressure. Hypokalaemia may be a clue to excessive liquorice ingestion as a cause of hypertension.

THYROTOXICOSIS

Hyperthyroidism may be a cause of hypertension. Although mean arterial pressure is not usually raised, systolic blood pressure and cardiac output may be significantly elevated. Other associated abnormalities include tachycardia and atrial arrhythmias. Thyroid hormones are thought to have direct stimulatory effects on the myocardium and also increase responses to sympathetic nervous system stimulation. The hypertension of thyrotoxicosis usually resolves following treatment of the thyroid condition. However, there is some evidence that people with treated hyperthyroidism are at higher cardiovascular risk than the general population.

RARE MONOGENIC SYNDROMES

LIDDLE'S SYNDROME

Liddle's syndrome is an autosomal dominant condition characterized by early-onset hypertension and hypokalaemia associated with low circulating renin and aldosterone levels.[1] It is caused by mutations in the genes encoding the β and γ subunits of the mineralocorticoid-dependent epithelial sodium channel, which result in constitutive (continuous) activation of the channel in the absence of mineralocorticoid, leading to increased sodium reabsorption and hypertension. The condition responds to the epithelial sodium channel blocker triamterene.

GLUCOCORTICOID-REMEDIABLE ALDOSTERONISM

Glucocorticoid-remediable aldosteronism is an autosomal dominant condition characterized by low-renin hypertension and elevated aldosterone levels.[2] A chromosomal translocation between the genes encoding aldosterone synthase and 11β-hydroxylase, two enzymes involved in steroid biosynthesis, results in a loss of the normal secretory control processes, such that ACTH rather than angiotensin II stimulates aldosterone secretion. There is also a loss of negative feedback of circulating aldosterone levels on ACTH secretion, leading to excessive aldosterone levels. The excessive mineralocorticoid activity leads to salt and water retention and hypertension.

The abnormal ACTH secretion may be suppressed by the administration of glucocorticoids such as dexamethasone, which is the treatment of choice in this condition and results in control of the hypertension. There are around 200 known cases of this condition worldwide.

APPARENT MINERALOCORTICOID EXCESS

This autosomal, recessively inherited condition results in hypertension with high circulating cortisol levels and low renin and aldosterone levels.[3] A mutation in the gene encoding 11β-hydroxysteroid dehydrogenase results in a reduction in the normal conversion of cortisol to cortisone. Unlike cortisone, cortisol is able to act as a potent agonist at the mineralocorticoid receptor, leading to hypertension. Clinically this syndrome resembles primary hyperaldosteronism; however, the aldosterone level is characteristically low. The 24-hour urinary cortisol levels are characteristically high.

The condition responds to high doses of spironolactone or amiloride. Dexamethasone is also given to suppress endogenous cortisol secretion.

GORDON'S SYNDROME (PSEUDOHYPOALDOSTERONISM TYPE II)

This autosomal dominant condition is characterized by:

- early-onset low-renin hypertension
- increased renal sodium reabsorption
- hyperkalaemia
- hyperchloraemia.

Two genes with mutations causing this condition have recently been identified as the with no lysine K (WNK) kinase genes WNK1 and WNK4.[4] The abnormalities are reversed by therapy with thiazide diuretics.

OTHER MONOGENIC SYNDROMES

A mutation in the mineralocorticoid receptor causing early-onset hypertension that is severely exacerbated in pregnancy due to increased progesterone levels has been described. This mutation is extremely rare, with fewer than 10 cases described worldwide (see

Hypertension in pregnancy, p. 203). Hypertension and brachydactyly is an autosomal dominant condition that has been localized to a gene on chromosome 12. Monogenic syndromes are also responsible for some cases of phaeochromocytoma (see p. 45). The search for other mutations that may be related to hypertension is ongoing.

REFERENCES

1. Liddle GW, Bledsoe T, Coppage WS. A familial renal disorder simulating primary aldosteronism but with negligible aldosterone secretion. Trans Assoc Physicians 1966; 76: 199–213.
2. Sutherland DJ, Ruse JL, Laidlaw JC. Hypertension, increased aldosterone secretion and low plasma renin activity relieved by dexamethasone. Can Med Assoc J 1966; 95: 1109–1119.
3. Stewart PM, Corrie JE, Shackleton CH, et al. Syndrome of apparent mineralocorticoid excess. A defect in the cortisol–cortisone shuttle. J Clin Invest 1988; 82: 340–349
4. Wilson FH, Disse-Nicodeme S, Choate KA, et al. Human hypertension caused by mutations in WNK kinases. Science 2001; 293: 1107–1112.

CLINICAL
ASSESSMENT OF
HYPERTENSION

HISTORY AND EXAMINATION

SIGNS AND SYMPTOMS

Essential hypertension is usually an asymptomatic condition and is often detected only by chance during routine measurement of blood pressure. This emphasizes the importance of regular blood pressure checks, especially in patients with borderline hypertension, in those with other cardiovascular risk factors, and in older individuals, amongst whom hypertension is particularly common. Key points to cover during history taking include the following.

- The duration of hypertension where possible; ask about the results of any previous blood pressure checks (e.g. attendance at an earlier clinic or insurance medical).
- Raised blood pressure in pregnancy or pre-eclampsia.
- Family history of hypertension or cardiovascular disease (usually a first-degree relative aged less than 60 at the time of diagnosis).
- Smoking habit, diabetes mellitus and hypercholesterolaemia, to assess overall cardiovascular risk.
- Lifestyle factors such as alcohol intake, levels of physical activity, dietary habits (including salt intake), and fresh fruit and vegetable consumption.
- Consider features suggestive of a secondary cause for high blood pressure (see *Pointers to secondary hypertension*, p. 65).
- Current and previous drug therapy, and drug intolerances or allergies; ask specifically about use of the oral contraceptive pill in younger women.

There is often little to find on examination, except perhaps evidence of end-organ damage (see *End-organ damage*, p. 67), and it is important that all hypertensive patients are screened for this. Nevertheless, a thorough physical examination is required at the initial consultation and should include the following.

- Height and weight, with body mass index calculated using the formula weight (kg)/height (m)^2.
- Measurement of the blood pressure (see *Measurement of blood pressure*, p. 73).
- Cardiovascular system examination should focus on evidence of valvular heart disease, heart failure, cardiac arrhythmia, peripheral arterial insufficiency, bruits or radio-femoral delay.
- The kidneys should be examined carefully for apparent bruits or masses.
- Examination of the central nervous system should be performed, looking for any clinical signs of cerebrovascular damage, and the appearance of both retinas on fundoscopy should be noted.

Individuals with malignant hypertension or secondary hypertension may experience a number of symptoms such as headache (Table 2.1), and signs due to the underlying condition may be evident.

POINTERS TO SECONDARY HYPERTENSION

Although the majority of hypertensive patients will have essential hypertension, an underlying cause can be identified in a significant minority with so-called 'secondary hypertension' (see *Secondary hypertension*, p. 33). The exact proportion depends on patient selection and the rigour of investigation, but it is approximately 5–10% of all patients with hypertension. Therefore it is important to consider secondary hypertension when taking a history and examining a hypertensive patient. The following are pointers to a possible underlying cause (see also Table 2.1).

- Renovascular disease: elderly, male, cigarette smoker, atheromatous disease elsewhere, vascular bruits, renal impairment or a significant rise in creatinine during angiotensin-converting enzyme inhibitor treatment, drug-resistant hypertension.
- Phaeochromocytoma: a diverse range of clinical features including headache, palpitations, particularly labile blood pressure, heart failure in young individuals, and a paradoxical blood pressure increase with non-selective β-blocker therapy due to unopposed intense α-receptor-mediated vasoconstriction.
- Hyperaldosteronism: hypokalaemia.
- Cushing's disease: diabetes mellitus, obesity, typical appearance.

The enthusiasm with which a secondary cause is sought will depend on other factors, for example whether blood pressure control can be attained without the need for any further intervention, or whether the results of investigation (e.g. in renal artery stenosis) would alter management.

FEATURES OF MALIGNANT HYPERTENSION

Malignant or accelerated-phase hypertension refers to the combination of a raised blood pressure, usually markedly so but not always, and retinal haemorrhages or papilloedema. Headache is

TABLE 2.1 Features suggestive of secondary hypertension

Cause	Suggestive features	Specialist investigations
Renovascular disease	Elderly, male, smoker Widespread atherosclerosis Hyperkalaemia or rise in creatinine in response to ACE inhibitor	MAG3 captopril renogram Magnetic resonance angiography Renal artery angiography
Cushing's syndrome	Cushingoid appearance Muscle weakness, fatigue Hirsutism	Dexamethasone suppression test CT or MRI scan of abdomen Consider chest or head scan to exclude lung or pituitary tumour
Primary hyperaldosteronism	Spontaneous hypokalaemia Diuretic-induced hypokalaemia Family history	Erect and supine aldosterone : plasma renin activity ratio Salt load and 24-hour urine aldosterone CT or MRI scan of abdomen Venous sampling
Phaeochromocytoma	Anxiety, tachycardia Postural hypotension Episodic headache	24-hour urinary catecholamines Plasma catecholamines MIBG uptake scintigraphy CT or MRI of adrenals Venous sampling

ACE, angiotensin-converting enzyme; CT, computerized tomography; MRI, magnetic resonance imaging; MIBG, ^{131}I-metaiodobenzylguanidine.

common in malignant hypertension, and end-organ damage is usually striking.

- About 30% of patients with malignant hypertension present with cardiac failure and pulmonary oedema, owing to the combination of increased circulating volume, increased cardiac after-load, and functional impairment of the ischaemic left ventricle.
- Acute renal impairment occurs in the majority of patients with malignant hypertension and is virtually always associated with increased circulating fluid volume. In severe cases dialysis may be required, particularly when there is pre-existing renal disease, and the prognosis is better if renal size, assessed by ultrasonography, is normal. Microscopic appearances indicate renal ischaemia and acute tubular necrosis, along with characteristic features of hypertensive end-organ damage, including fibrinoid necrosis and hyaline arteriosclerosis.
- In some cases malignant hypertension can be associated with abdominal pain due to gastrointestinal ischaemia, and even intestinal and pancreatic infarction.
- Encephalopathy may also occur due to focal cerebral oedema secondary to impaired cerebral auto-regulation. The majority of encephalopathy patients present with headache, but up to a third may have delirium, hemiparesis, cortical visual loss, coma or seizures.

END-ORGAN DAMAGE

End-organ damage refers to a particular pattern of structural abnormalities that occur as a direct consequence of exposure to persistently high blood pressure. At the microscopic level, the resistance arterioles undergo remodelling characterized by smooth muscle hypertrophy and collagen deposition in the sub-endothelial space. These structural changes reduce vessel lumen, thus increasing systemic vascular resistance, and hence high blood pressure begets further increased blood pressure. The larger arteries dilate and become stiffer (arteriosclerosis). This can be detected by an increase in the pulse wave velocity and enhanced wave reflection. Both these factors lead to a relatively greater rise in aortic pressure compared with pressure in the arm, which further increases the left ventricular after-load and risk of stroke. In addition, large artery stiffening may more directly promote the development of atheroma, and thus may be an additional, independent risk factor for cardiovascular disease.

Many organs are protected from the effects of elevated systemic blood pressure by auto-regulation, which serves to maintain normal tissue blood flow, and when hypertension is slowly progressive there is a degree of adaptation to higher pressures. However, continuous exposure to elevated blood pressure ultimately leads to organ damage, most notably in the kidney, heart and brain.

HYPERTENSIVE NEPHROPATHY

Hypertensive nephropathy is associated with a gradual decline in creatinine clearance, and in cases of malignant hypertension acute renal failure can occur. Frank proteinuria is an important risk factor for subsequent renal failure and cardiovascular disease, and it is also correlated with overall mortality in hypertensive patients.

Microalbuminuria (defined as a urinary albumin excretion of 20–200 mg/L) is more common in hypertensive patients than in normotensive ones, and is considered to be a sensitive marker of early non-specific kidney damage. Microalbuminuria is more closely related to ambulatory blood pressure than to clinic pressure, and it also correlates with left ventricular mass and retinopathy. The treatment of hypertension also reduces or reverses microalbuminuria. These findings suggest that microalbuminuria may be a useful measure of end-organ damage and cardiovascular risk in hypertensive patients, which is supported by limited data from relatively small studies. However, data from large trials are lacking, and, at present, the true predictive value of microalbuminuria is uncertain. Nevertheless, the presence of microalbuminuria in a hypertensive patient should prompt a more detailed search for evidence of other organ damage.

Microscopic haematuria is also a marker of hypertensive renal damage, although it is less closely related to clinical outcome than is proteinuria. The renal morphological changes associated with essential hypertension include hyaline arteriosclerosis, focal glomerular obsolescence, and thickening of glomerular basement membranes. These renal abnormalities are associated with decreased glomerular filtration, red blood cell urinary casts, and in some cases persistent microscopic haematuria. Haematuria is also associated with

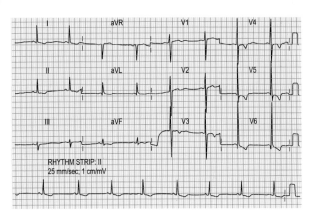

Fig. 2.1 Electrocardiogram of left ventricular hypertrophy. Note the increased voltages in lead I and the anterior chest leads, and the left ventricular strain pattern in the lateral chest leads.

some forms of renal parenchymal disease, and may, therefore, suggest an underlying cause for hypertension.

LEFT VENTRICULAR HYPERTROPHY

Cardiac end-organ response to sustained hypertension is concentric left ventricular hypertrophy, which may be detected in some cases by electrocardiography (Fig. 2.1), echocardiography or MRI scan. Chest radiography is a poor test for left ventricular hypertrophy (Fig. 2.2).

Together with an altered perfusion gradient due to higher ventricular pressure, left ventricular hypertrophy places increased demand on coronary blood supply and predisposes to myocardial ischaemia and microscopic foci of myocardial necrosis, which further impair cardiac performance.

Left ventricular hypertrophy is a poor prognostic indicator in hypertensive patients, irrespective of blood pressure itself, although it may regress if adequate blood pressure control is attained. Apart from perhaps β blockers, there seems to be little difference in the capacity of various anti-hypertensive drugs to induce regression for given reductions in peripheral pressures. Clearly hypertension can also promote the development of heart failure, angina and myocardial infarction.

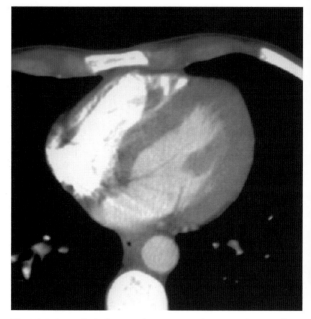

Fig. 2.2 Left ventricular hypertrophy. A computed tomography scan of the chest, showing marked left ventricular hypertrophy in this 19-year-old patient with malignant hypertension. In contrast, his chest radiograph appeared normal.

Disruption of normal cerebral blood flow often manifests insidiously and predisposes to progressive cortical loss, manifesting as non-Alzheimer's dementia. Hypertension is also a potent risk factor for cerebrovascular disease. In malignant hypertension, rapid elevation of blood pressure can overwhelm cerebral auto-regulation mechanisms, typically where mean arterial pressure exceeds 180 mmHg. This can cause cerebral arteriolar vasodilatation, oedema and microhaemorrhages, presenting clinically as delirium or acute encephalopathy (hypertensive encephalopathy).

HYPERTENSIVE RETINOPATHY

Hypertensive retinopathy reflects the abnormal microvascular responses to hypertension occurring elsewhere in the body.

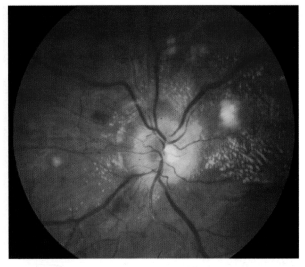

Fig. 2.3 Hypertensive retinopathy. Fundus of a 24-year-old woman with malignant hypertension, illustrating grade IV hypertensive retinopathy. Note the presence of papilloedema, cotton wool spots and haemorrhages.

The features of hypertensive retinopathy can include the appearance of:

- silver wiring
- arteriovenous nipping
- cotton wool spots
- flame-shaped haemorrhages
- macular oedema
- macular star or ring of exudates
- disc oedema
- (ultimately) papilloedema (Fig. 2.3).

Exudation and papilloedema are thought to arise from accumulation of axoplasmatic debris due to ischaemia-induced obstruction of axoplasmic flow.

The severity of hypertensive retinopathy can be described by several grading systems, and the one endorsed by the British Hypertension Society is the Keith, Wagener and Barker classification

TABLE 2.2 Grades of hypertensive retinopathy

Grade	Features
Grade I	Mild narrowing or sclerosis of the retinal arterioles No symptoms, good general health
Grade II	Moderate to marked sclerosis of the retinal arterioles Exaggerated light reflex Venous compression at arteriovenous crossings ('A–V nipping') No symptoms, good general health
Grade III	Retinal oedema, cotton wool spots Haemorrhages Sclerosis and spastic lesions of retinal arterioles Often symptomatic
Grade IV (malignant hypertension)	All of the above Optic disc oedema (papilloedema) Symptomatic Cardiac and renal function often impaired; reduced survival

(From Dodson et al 1996,[1] with permission.)

(Table 2.2). Adequate treatment often leads to a complete reversal of retinopathy.

REFERENCE

1. Dodson PM, Lip GY, Eames SM, et al. Hypertensive retinopathy: a review of existing classification systems and a suggestion for a simplified grading system. J Hum Hypertens 1996; 10: 93–98.

MEASUREMENT OF BLOOD PRESSURE

TECHNIQUE OF MEASUREMENT

- Usually blood pressure is measured in the brachial artery after 5 minutes' seated rest.
- It is important to use the correct size of cuff: the bladder should enclose 80% of the arm.
- The cuff should be applied securely to the upper arm, with the bladder centred over the brachial artery; further details of the manual technique are given in Box 2.1.
- Usually at least two measurements should be taken, and if they vary widely, a third.
- The patient should be relaxed and comfortable, and should not talk while blood pressure is being assessed.
- Blood pressure should be recorded to the nearest 2 mmHg to avoid digit preference.

During the initial assessment, blood pressure should be measured in both arms in all hypertensive patients. This is of particular importance when the clinical history suggests coarctation or other

---

Box 2.1 Measuring blood pressure

- Support the arm in a horizontal position at the level of the mid-sternum.
- Next inflate the cuff until the brachial artery pulse disappears. This provides an estimate of systolic pressure and ensures that the cuff is correctly seated on the arm.
- Deflate the cuff, then re-inflate to 30 mmHg above estimated systolic pressure. Deflate at 2–3 mmHg per second and listen over the brachial artery for the first occurrence of repetitive tapping sounds (Korotkoff I), which equates to systolic pressure. Diastolic pressure is conventionally taken at the disappearance of sounds (Korotkoff V).*

*If the sounds do not disappear, as is occasionally the case (e.g. in some pregnant women), muffling of the sounds (Korotkoff IV) is taken instead: this should be noted.
Full details for measuring blood pressure are available from http://www.abdn.ac.uk/medical/bhs/booklet/intro.htm.

serious aortic pathology (e.g. dissection). However, in general it does not matter which arm blood pressure is measured in, as long as pressure does not differ greatly between the two arms (less than 15 mmHg). If there is a significant difference, then the arm with the higher reading should be used and this fact noted.

During the initial assessment, it is also important to check for postural hypotension. Blood pressure should be measured with the patient lying down and again after 2–3 minutes of standing. If there is no significant drop (less than 15 mmHg), then this need only be repeated at future visits if symptoms suggest postural hypotension, which is more common in the elderly and in those taking vasodilating agents such as α blockers.

To provide an accurate diagnosis of hypertension, two readings of blood pressure should be obtained on three separate occasions, usually about 1 month apart. In those with high-normal blood pressure the period of observation may be longer, with more readings being made. Conversely, the observation period should be reduced in patients with clear evidence of end-organ damage or accelerated (malignant) hypertension, so that treatment can be initiated sooner.

> ⚠️ **Failure to assess blood pressure on more than one occasion greatly increases the over-diagnosis of hypertension, leading to inappropriate treatment and worry.**

OBESE PATIENTS AND CHILDREN

Unless the correct size of cuff is used, blood pressure recordings are inaccurate. Although using a cuff that is too large has little or no effect on measured blood pressure, using a cuff that is too small (i.e. the bladder does not encompass 80% of the arm) leads to an over-estimation of blood pressure.

> ⚠️ **The most frequent cause of incorrect blood pressure measurement is an inappropriately small cuff: if in doubt use a larger cuff. Larger cuffs should be available for use in obese patients, and small (paediatric) cuffs for children (Fig. 2.4).**

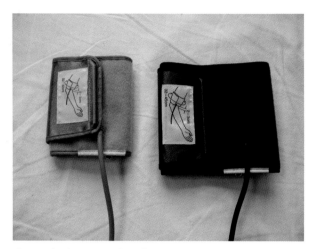

Fig. 2.4 Blood pressure cuffs. Different sizes of blood pressure cuff are available for use in obese adults, in normal adults and older children, and in infants. It is important to select the correct cuff size for an individual patient to avoid inaccurate readings.

AUTOMATED SPHYGMOMANOMETERS

For nearly 100 years, mercury sphygmomanometers have been the gold standard for non-invasive assessment of blood pressure. Largely unfounded concerns over mercury and the desire to remove operator error have led to the development of automated sphygmomanometers. There are two basic types:

● oscillometric sphygmomanometers
● auscultatory sphygmomanometers.

Oscillometric machines are more commonly used, especially in the home situation. They rely on oscillations in the bladder—induced by blood pulsating through a partly occluded brachial artery—to estimate blood pressure; maximal oscillation occurs when cuff pressure equals brachial artery mean pressure. Although often easier to use, there is no real advantage to automated sphygmomanometers over traditional mercury column devices in everyday clinical practice, and they may even be worse if no or inappropriate training has been given. Nevertheless, automated devices do remove digit preference and provide a degree of measurement standardization, and they are thus often used in the clinical trial setting.

Important: Oscillometric sphygmomanometers are thought to be less reliable in the elderly and in patients with atrial fibrillation. Only devices validated by the British Hypertension Society should be used (see http://www.hyp.ac.uk/bhsinfo/bpmindex.html for a list).

ANEROID DEVICES

Aneroid devices are in widespread use. However, they require regular calibration, which is rarely undertaken, and large swings in the needle during measurements can make accurate determination of blood pressure impossible. Indeed, standard aneroid devices do not meet the British Hypertension Society validation criteria. For these reasons, aneroid devices are probably best avoided unless a simple rough estimate of blood pressure is required (e.g. in an emergency situation).

AMBULATORY BLOOD PRESSURE MONITORING

In recent years there has been a great deal of interest in 24-hour ambulatory blood pressure monitoring (ABPM), and there are now several validated devices available (see http://www.hyp.ac.uk/bhsinfo/bpmindex.html for a list). However, ABPM is not necessary for either diagnosis or management in the majority of hypertensive patients. Indeed, the risk associated with hypertension and benefits of therapy have been almost exclusively established using seated clinic pressure recordings.

Data suggest that ABPM values correlate more closely with surrogate measures such as left ventricular hypertrophy and carotid intima media thickness, but virtually no outcome data concerning ABPM exist. Nevertheless, ABPM can be useful in selected patients, such as:

- those with particularly labile pressures
- those with high clinic recordings but no evidence of end-organ damage.

Average ABPM values are invariably lower that those recorded in the clinic, and thus an individual with a daytime ABPM average of 150/100 mmHg is probably at more risk than one with the same clinic pressure. Therefore thresholds for therapy and targets need to be lowered when ABPM values are used (about 10/5 mmHg lower).

Usually the average daytime value is used from ABPM to guide management decisions. However, it has been suggested that the lack of a nocturnal dip in blood pressure may be of prognostic significance (Fig. 2.5).

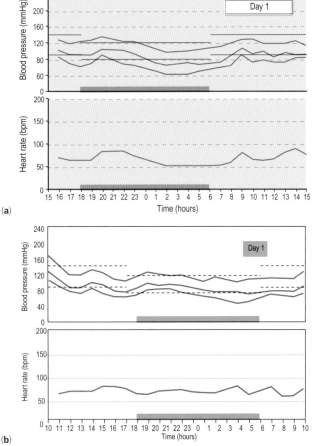

Fig. 2.5 Four 24-hour ambulatory blood pressure monitoring (ABPM) traces (hourly averages): (**a**) normal blood pressure; (**b**) white coat hypertension—initial readings are high but the blood pressure then settles into the normal range; (**c**) hypertension with normal night-time dipping of blood pressure; and (**d**) hypertension with loss of the normal night-time dipping of blood pressure (i.e. 'non-dipper').

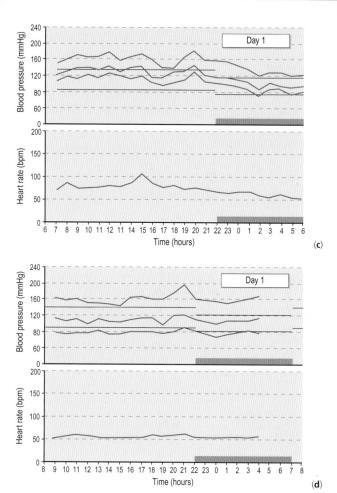

Fig. 2.5 *Continued*

HOME MONITORING OF BLOOD PRESSURE

A wealth of automated sphygmomanometers is now available directly to the general public, although not all have been validated. Provided that patients are correctly using a well-maintained, validated automated sphygmomanometer, then home monitoring is generally reliable. Indeed, home monitoring can shorten the time taken for diagnosis and to achieve target pressure once therapy has been initiated. However, as with ambulatory monitoring, home values are invariably lower than those obtained in the clinic and thresholds should be adjusted accordingly.

INVESTIGATIONS

There are a number of standard investigations that are appropriate for most hypertensive individuals. These are listed in Box 2.2 together with some more detailed investigations that are relevant for selected patients, usually to investigate secondary causes of hypertension. A chest X-ray is not part of the routine assessment of hypertensive patients. Rather, it is reserved for those patients in whom symptoms or physical signs suggest involvement of the respiratory system, particularly where pulmonary oedema is suspected.

LABORATORY INVESTIGATIONS

- A full lipid profile (total cholesterol, LDL and HDL cholesterol, and triglycerides) and glucose should be performed in all patients as a screening tool to estimate each individual's coronary heart disease risk.
- This is most commonly performed in the non-fasting state, which is probably adequate for the majority of patients.
- It should be repeated in the fasting state if diabetes is suspected or cholesterol levels suggest treatment is indicated.

Uric acid is not measured consistently in the assessment of all hypertensive patients, largely because debate persists as to whether raised serum urate is an independent cardiovascular risk factor or simply a marker of other factors. Nevertheless, measurement of serum urate concentrations may be important in identifying those

---

Box 2.2 Routine and selected investigations in patients with hypertension

Routinely indicated
Urinalysis for protein, blood and glucose
Serum urea, creatinine and electrolytes
Blood glucose
Serum total : HDL cholesterol ratio
Electrocardiography

Indicated in selected patients
Echocardiography
Urine microscopy and culture
Chest X-ray
Urinary catecholamine metabolites
Plasma renin and aldosterone

patients with particularly high concentrations, who may be exposed to a greater risk of gout, especially if thiazide diuretic treatment is contemplated.

ELECTROCARDIOGRAPHY

A 12-lead electrocardiogram (ECG) is recommended for all patients with hypertension. This serves as a crude screen for left ventricular hypertrophy (see Fig. 2.1, p. 69), which is an important independent risk factor in hypertensive patients. Moreover, a routine ECG will identify any underlying cardiac dysrhythmia, and in some cases may identify coexistent myocardial ischaemia.

ECHOCARDIOGRAPHY

An echocardiogram is most useful for confirming or refuting the presence of left ventricular hypertrophy where there is some degree of suspicion. Left ventricular hypertrophy is an important independent marker of increased cardiovascular risk in hypertension, and its presence may be suggested by findings on:

- physical examination, including left para-sternal heave
- chest X-ray
- the ECG (e.g. high left ventricular voltages, S–T segment depression and dysrhythmia).

In addition, echocardiography is particularly helpful in patients with borderline or resistant hypertension, when the presence of left ventricular hypertrophy would alter the treatment plan.

SPECIFIC INVESTIGATIONS FOR SECONDARY CAUSES OF HYPERTENSION

In evaluating the hypertensive patient, patient characteristics, symptoms and/or physical signs, laboratory investigations, and response to treatment may all suggest an underlying cause (Box 2.2). The nature of any further investigations will be directed by the suspected underlying cause. In most cases, this is probably most appropriately directed by a hypertension specialist, because interpretation can be difficult and the precision of the test depends on local expertise. Further details of the specific investigations are provided in *Secondary hypertension* (p. 33).

CHAPTER 3

TREATMENT OF HYPERTENSION

RISK ASSESSMENT

Large, population-based cohort studies have demonstrated a strong association between the level of blood pressure and cardiovascular risk. This relationship is graded and continuous, with no apparent threshold of risk. There is a similar relationship between blood pressure and all-cause mortality.[1] The relationship is stronger for systolic blood pressure than for diastolic pressure, and it is consistent in patients with and without evidence of atheromatous disease. Recently, a number of studies have emphasized the importance of pulse pressure (systolic blood pressure minus diastolic blood pressure) as a predictor of risk, especially in patients over the age of 60 years.[2,3]

The population risk of cardiovascular disease attributable to hypertension is enormous. High blood pressure causes:

- approximately 35% of all cardiovascular events[4]
- approximately 50% of all congestive cardiac failure
- 25% of all premature deaths.

However, the absolute risk for an individual depends on the presence or absence of a number of associated risk factors and also on the presence or absence of target organ damage, especially left ventricular hypertrophy, which is an established independent risk factor for mortality. Additional risk factors can be broadly classified as those that are non-modifiable (Box 3.1) and those that are modifiable (Box 3.2). In addition, a number of new potential risk factors are emerging (Box 3.3), although the influence of these factors on total cardiovascular risk remains to be established and quantified.

Because the risk of cardiovascular morbidity and mortality in patients with hypertension depends more on the sum of risk factors than on actual blood pressure, to predict the prognosis of individual patients it is necessary to evaluate their absolute risk of cardiovascular disease. A number of methods are in use to calculate the risk of cardiovascular disease in a patient with hypertension (Box 3.4).[7] These methods are based on entering data on a patient's modifiable and non-modifiable risk factors, for which strong evidence exists for a relationship to cardiovascular disease and benefits from modification.

The British Hypertension Society guidelines for 2004 recommend that in addition to anti-hypertensive therapy to reduce blood pressure, other drug therapy to reduce cardiovascular risk should also be considered.[13]

- Aspirin is recommended for the secondary prevention of cardiovascular disease.

Box 3.1 Non-modifiable risk factors that influence prognosis in hypertension

Age
Risk increases with increasing age. This could be partly due to increases in hypertension and diabetes that are associated with age.

Sex
Incidence of myocardial infarction is greater for men and lower in women until after the menopause.

Ethnicity and race
Incidence of cardiovascular disease varies among ethnicities and races. This could be associated with genetic differences and also differences in risk factors. Afro-Caribbean people have an increased incidence of hypertension and are at increased risk of stroke.

Family history
Family history of premature heart disease increases the relative risk in family members.

Box 3.2 Modifiable risk factors that influence prognosis in hypertension

Systolic and diastolic blood pressure
There is good evidence that blood pressure control reduces cardiovascular risk irrespective of the anti-hypertensive agent used: the lower the blood pressure, the lower the risk.

Pulse pressure
Although anti-hypertensive agents have differing effects on pulse pressure, no randomized trials have been conducted showing greater benefits from drugs producing larger decreases in pulse pressure.

Cholesterol
Meta-analysis of recent studies shows that a 0.6-mmol/L decrease in total cholesterol is associated with a significant reduction in ischaemic heart disease.[5]

Continued

Box 3.2 Modifiable risk factors that influence prognosis in hypertension—cont'd

Triglycerides
The relationship between raised triglycerides and cardiovascular risk is less well established. Some studies have shown benefit from reduction of triglycerides in patients with established coronary artery disease. However, these trials also raised HDL cholesterol, making the results of such studies difficult to interpret.

Smoking
Smoking is a major risk factor for cardiovascular disease. No randomized trials have examined the effects of smoking cessation on cardiovascular outcome. However, observational studies suggest that the cardiovascular risk profiles of smokers become similar to those of non-smokers after approximately 1–3 years.

Diabetes mellitus
Diabetes mellitus is a major risk factor for cardiovascular disease (see *Diabetes and hypertension*, p. 169). Good glycaemic control decreases the development of microvascular complications in both type 1 and type 2 diabetes. However, glycaemic control has no effect on macrovascular disease. The UK Prospective Diabetes Study showed that tight blood pressure control produces more benefit in terms of macrovascular disease than tight glycaemic control.

Physical inactivity
Meta-analysis showed a 1.6-fold increase in coronary artery disease in those with decreased physical activity relative to control subjects.[6] However, no trials of increasing physical activity in relation to cardiovascular outcome have been performed.

Obesity
There is a strong positive association between increased body mass index and cardiovascular disease. Much of this increased risk may be due to clustering of other cardiovascular risk factors, including:

- hypertension
- diabetes

Continued

Box 3.2 Modifiable risk factors that influence prognosis in hypertension—cont'd

- hypercholesterolaemia
- insulin resistance.

No trials on the effect of weight loss on cardiovascular outcome have been performed, although weight loss does slow the onset of type 2 diabetes.

Left ventricular hypertrophy
The prevalence of left ventricular hypertrophy is between 16 and 23% in individuals with hypertension. Left ventricular hypertrophy has been shown to significantly increase the risk of cardiovascular disease. Drug treatment can decrease left ventricular hypertrophy, but no trials have been performed to support an association between decreased left ventricular hypertrophy and improved cardiovascular outcome.

Microalbuminuria
Evidence of microalbuminuria as a risk factor for cardiovascular disease in hypertensive individuals is less strong than in those with diabetes. Again, anti-hypertensive medication has been shown to decrease microalbuminuria, but as yet this has not been correlated with improved cardiovascular outcome.

Uric acid
Up to one-third of hypertensive persons have raised uric acid levels. This is probably a marker for cardiovascular disease rather than a cause. No trials have shown that decreasing uric acid improves cardiovascular outcome.

Box 3.3 Emerging risk factors that may influence prognosis in hypertensive patients

Fibrinogen
Homocysteine
C-reactive protein levels
Low HDL
Albumin
von Willebrand factor
High-risk genotypes
Lipoprotein (a)

Box 3.4 Methods for cardiovascular risk assessment in hypertensive patients

Framingham risk equation[8]
Dundee coronary risk disc[9]
PROCAM risk function[10]
SCORE system[11]
PRECARD system[12]

- Aspirin is also recommended for patients over the age of 50 years whose blood pressure is controlled to less than 150/90 mmHg and who have a 10-year cardiovascular disease risk of at least 20% (measured using the new Joint British Societies' cardiovascular disease risk chart).
- Statin therapy is recommended for patients up to the age of at least 80 years with hypertension, a total cholesterol of at least 3.5 mmol/L, and a 10-year cardiovascular disease risk of at least 20%. The dose of statin should be titrated upwards to achieve target cholesterol levels.

REFERENCES

1. Antikainen R, Jousilahti P, Tuomilehto J. Systolic blood pressure, isolated systolic hypertension and risk of coronary heart disease, strokes, cardiovascular disease and all-cause mortality in the middle-aged population. J Hypertens 1998; 16(5): 577–583.
2. Rutan GH, Kuller LH, Neaton JD, et al. Mortality associated with diastolic hypertension and isolated systolic hypertension among men screened for the Multiple Risk Factor Intervention Trial. Circulation 1988; 77(3): 504–514.
3. Franklin SS, Gustin IVW, Wong ND, et al. Hemodynamic patterns of age-related changes in blood pressure: The Framingham Heart Study. Circulation 1997; 96: 308–315.
4. Kannel WB. Blood pressure as a cardiovascular risk factor: prevention and treatment. JAMA 1996; 275(20): 1571–1576.
5. Law MR, Wald NJ, Thompson SG. By how much and how quickly does reduction in serum cholesterol concentration lower risk of ischaemic heart disease? Br Med J 1994; 308: 367–372.
6. Berlin JA, Colditz GA. A meta-analysis of physical activity in the prevention of coronary heart disease. Am J Epidemiol 1990; 132: 612–628.
7. Haq IU, Ramsay LE, Jackson PR, et al. Prediction of coronary risk for primary prevention of coronary heart disease: a comparison of methods. Q J Med 1999; 92(7): 379–385.

8. Wilson PW, D'Agostino RB, Levy D, et al. Prediction of coronary heart disease using risk factor categories. Circulation 1998; 97: 1837–1847.
9. Tunstall-Pedoe H. The Dundee coronary risk-disk for management of change in risk factors. Br Med J 1991; 303: 744–747.
10. Assmann G, Cullen P, Schulte H, et al. The Münster Heart Study (PROCAM): results of follow-up at 8 years. Eur Heart J 1998; 19(Suppl A): A2–A11.
11. Conroy RM, Pyorala K, Fitzgerald AP, et al. Estimation of ten-year risk of fatal cardiovascular disease in Europe: the SCORE project. Eur Heart J 2003; 24; 987–1003.
12. Thomsen TF, Davidsen M, Ibsen H, et al. A new method for CHD prediction and prevention based on regional risk scores and randomized clinical trials: PRECARD and the Copenhagen Risk Score. J Cardiovasc Risk 2001; 8: 291–297.
13. Williams B, Poulter NR, Brown MJ, et al. Guidelines for management of hypertension: report of the Fourth Working Party of the British Hypertension Society, 2004—BHS IV. J Hum Hypertens 2004; 18(3): 139–185.

LIFESTYLE MEASURES

> **Box 3.5 Lifestyle issues targeted by the national service framework for coronary heart disease**
>
> Reducing smoking
> Increasing physical activity
> Promoting healthy eating habits
> Reducing overweight and obesity

Standards 1–4 of the UK national service framework for coronary heart disease (CHD) are focused on:

- the reduction of CHD in the general population
- preventing cardiovascular disease in high-risk patients.

To this end, a number of lifestyle factors are being addressed by the NHS, working in partnership with local authorities, to produce local policies on a number of lifestyle issues (Box 3.5).

SALT RESTRICTION

Early humans evolved on a low-salt diet (20–40 mmol of sodium per day), and thus modern humans are adapted to the conservation of salt in the diet. With the introduction of more salt into the diet of modern humans, there is the requirement to excrete sodium loads of 10–20 times higher than the physiological needs.

Current consumption of sodium in the UK averages 140–150 mmol/day, although the physiological requirement is approximately 8–10 mmol/day. Early data from the 1940s, in the era before anti-hypertensive drugs, demonstrated that the Kempner low-salt diet is effective in the management of malignant hypertension.

EPIDEMIOLOGICAL DATA

Epidemiological evidence for a positive correlation between salt and blood pressure is derived from population-based studies. However, there were a number of methodological problems with such studies, and many were too small to demonstrate any clear association. An overview of 14 studies in 16 different populations demonstrated a highly significant positive association of sodium with both systolic and diastolic blood pressure; this association was higher in women than in men.[1]

To date, the largest study undertaken investigating the association between sodium and blood pressure is the INTERSALT study.[2] This study included data from over 10 000 men and women, aged 20–59 years, from 52 populations in 32 countries. Across the various populations, those with the sodium intake lower by 100 mmol/day had a decrease in the age-associated rise in systolic blood pressure of 7 mmHg and in diastolic blood pressure of 6 mmHg.

GENETICS: SALT SENSITIVITY

The relationship between salt and water intake and blood pressure is heterogeneous among individuals, such that they can be classified into two groups:

- salt-sensitive
- salt-resistant.

Two rare monogenic forms of hypertension are known to be salt-sensitive:

- glucocorticoid-remediable aldosteronism
- apparent mineralocorticoid excess.

Furthermore, a number of genes have been implicated in the relationship between salt and water intake and resultant blood pressure levels, including:

- α-adducin
- angiotensinogen
- angiotensin-converting enzyme (ACE).

CONTROLLED TRIALS OF SODIUM RESTRICTION

Randomized controlled trials in both hypertensive and normotensive individuals have shown systolic blood pressure falls of 6 mmHg following restriction of sodium intake from 170 to 70–90 mmol/day.[3] Although there were some initial concerns about the safety of moderate sodium restriction, these have not been substantiated.[4]

The Trial of Non-pharmacological Intervention in the Elderly (TONE) demonstrated that elderly, overweight hypertensive individuals could significantly reduce their need for anti-hypertensive medication by sodium restriction of 40 mmol/day.[5]

The Dietary Approaches to Stop Hypertension (DASH) trial provided participants with three levels of sodium intake:

- high (over 141 mmol/day)
- intermediate (106 mmol/day)
- low (64 mmol/day).

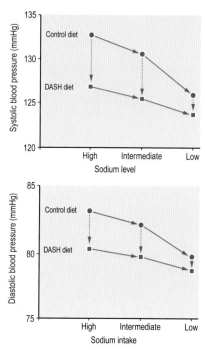

Fig. 3.1 Sodium restriction and blood pressure. In the Dietary Approaches to Stop Hypertension (DASH) trial, sodium restriction reduced blood pressure in a dose-dependent fashion. (From Sacks et al © 2001,[6] Massachusetts Medical Society. All rights reserved.)

These levels were verified using 24-hour urinary sodium determination. Not only did sodium restriction decrease blood pressure, but there was also a clear dose–response relationship (Fig. 3.1).[6]

CARDIOVASCULAR DISEASE

A number of observational studies have linked a high sodium intake with increased cardiovascular risk.[7] However, there are as yet no randomized controlled trials to demonstrate that salt restriction reduces cardiovascular morbidity or mortality. Indeed, evidence from cohort studies is conflicting, with some studies demonstrating benefit and some an increased cardiovascular risk.[8]

SALT RESTRICTION AND ANTI-HYPERTENSIVE THERAPY

Moderate salt restriction has been shown to augment the hypotensive effect of a number of anti-hypertensive agents including diuretics, β blockers and ACE inhibitors. In addition, two large studies, TONE and DASH, demonstrated that requirements for anti-hypertensive medication could be reduced by dietary salt restriction.

WEIGHT LOSS

Hypertension and obesity are closely related, such that blood pressure rises with increasing body weight, resulting in the incidence of hypertension being approximately 50% among obese individuals. Indeed, in population-based studies, weight or body mass index (BMI) is predictive of blood pressure,[9] and data from the Framingham study suggest that obesity or recent weight gain may account for 70% of new-onset hypertension. Obesity, therefore, is a major factor in the development of increased blood pressure.

In addition, obesity and hypertension occur together frequently as part of the metabolic syndrome, a combination of risk factors for cardiovascular disease that also include insulin resistance and dyslipidaemia (low HDL cholesterol and raised triglycerides). More than 20% of US adults have the metabolic syndrome.

Over the past decade there has been a marked increase in the prevalence of both obesity and the metabolic syndrome, with the alarming prediction that by 2015 more than 40% of the US population will be obese in terms of having a BMI of over 30 kg/m^2. Because obesity and the metabolic syndrome are major risk factors for cardiovascular disease, this has enormous implications for the future.

RELATIONSHIP BETWEEN OBESITY AND HYPERTENSION

The role of obesity in the pathophysiology of hypertension is unclear but may involve a number of factors (Box 3.6).

Most recently, obesity has been shown to be particularly associated with an increase in pulse pressure, suggesting that obesity may mediate hypertension via an increase in large arterial stiffness.

There is clear evidence from clinical trials that weight loss is associated with a reduction in blood pressure.[10] It has also been

Box 3.6 Factors involved in obesity-related hypertension

Body fat distribution : abdominal obesity, increased waist–hip ratio
Risk factor clustering : metabolic syndrome
Haemodynamics : increased blood volume, increased peripheral vascular resistance
Salt sensitivity : increased sodium intake
Increased sympathetic nervous system activity
Increased arterial stiffness
Endothelial dysfunction

Box 3.7 Benefits of weight reduction in hypertensive individuals

Decreased blood pressure
Decreased requirement for anti-hypertensive therapy
Improvement in lipid profile
Improved glucose sensitivity
Decreased arterial stiffness
Decreased left ventricular load

shown that this benefit persists relative to a control group who gain weight over the same period, even if the weight loss is not sustained. Augmented effects on blood pressure reduction are obtained if weight loss is accompanied by:

● decreased alcohol consumption
● decreased sodium intake
● increased fish consumption
● moderate exercise.

Overall, weight reduction can lead to a reduction of blood pressure of approximately 7/5 mmHg.[11]

In addition to blood pressure reduction, weight loss is associated with a number of other benefits in terms of reduced cardiovascular risk (Box 3.7).

EXERCISE

PHYSICAL INACTIVITY AND BLOOD PRESSURE

There is strong observational evidence to support a link between low physical activity and an increased incidence of hypertension.

However, many observational studies fail to control for other factors associated with hypertension between the active and inactive subject groups.

According to the national service framework for CHD (March 2000), 60% of men and 70% of women in the UK are considered to be physically inactive, which is associated with an approximate doubling of the risk of CHD.[12]

EXERCISE AND BLOOD PRESSURE

Over 50 controlled trials have examined the effect of exercise on blood pressure. A number of quantitative meta-analyses have been performed incorporating these trials. The results have included effects of aerobic exercise on blood pressure in both hypertensive and normotensive individuals, in women, and in older adults. In addition, the type of exercise has also been studied.

All studies have demonstrated significant decreases in both systolic and diastolic blood pressure, with the exception of diastolic blood pressure in older adults, which was not significantly reduced. Effects are greatest in hypertensive patients and are independent of changes in weight (Fig. 3.2).[13]

There is considerable debate as to the most effective type of exercise and its duration. However, overall it would appear that at least 2 hours/week of moderate-intensity exercise is necessary to achieve a clinically relevant benefit in terms of blood pressure.[13] Meta-analysis suggests that blood pressure reduction at low levels of exercise intensity is proportional to the duration of exercise. More evidence is needed as to the relative benefits of moderate versus vigorous exercise intensity.

Clinically, sedentary individuals should be encouraged to take moderate-intensity exercise such as brisk walking. Indeed, a 10-year study in 6017 normotensive sedentary Japanese men showed that simply walking to work reduces the incidence of hypertension. The study concluded that for every 26 men who walked to work for at least 21 minutes instead of 10 minutes or less, one case of hypertension would be prevented.[14]

EXERCISE AND REDUCTION IN CHD

There is a considerable body of evidence that increases in exercise reduce the risk of CHD, the greatest risk reductions being seen in

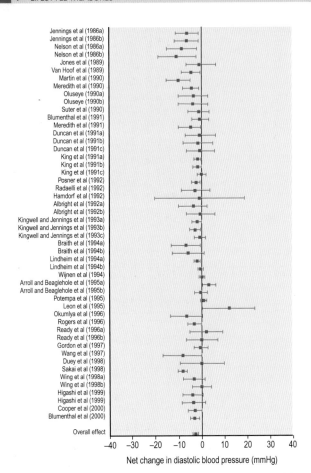

Fig. 3.2 Effects of exercise on diastolic blood pressure. This meta-analysis shows that diastolic blood pressure decreases with chronic exercise. (From Whelton et al 2002,[13] with permission.)

previously sedentary individuals who engage in moderate to vigorous physical activity. A 1999 study showed that walking 1.5 miles/day reduced the risk of CHD by 50% relative to men who walked only 0.25 miles or less; thus for each additional 0.5 miles' walk, the risk of CHD was reduced by 15%.[15]

Box 3.8 Contra-indications to exercise

Absolute contra-indications
Acute ischaemia
Certain arrhythmias
Infections

Relative contra-indications (at the physician's clinical judgement)
Systolic blood pressure > 200 mmHg or diastolic blood pressure > 115 mmHg
Valvular heart disease
Advanced congestive cardiac failure
Left ventricular aneurysm
Severe electrolyte imbalance

CONTRA-INDICATIONS TO EXERCISE

There is some concern as to the risk of a cardiac event immediately after exercise. Studies in patients post myocardial infarction show that although 4–7% of events occurred within 1 hour of vigorous physical activity, the absolute risk of myocardial infarction was only 6 per 100 000 middle-aged men per year (Box 3.8 lists contra-indications to exercise).

ALCOHOL RESTRICTION

ALCOHOL AND BLOOD PRESSURE

Many epidemiological studies have demonstrated a direct relationship between alcohol intake and hypertension, especially if the average alcohol intake exceeds two drinks per day. Indeed, population studies worldwide show a clear, consistent relationship between the amount of alcohol drunk, levels of blood pressure, and the prevalence of hypertension.

- The relationship holds true for men and women across all ethnic groups and appears to be independent of the type of alcohol consumed.
- The relationship is linear throughout the range of consumption. Although some earlier trials suggested a J-shaped association with blood pressure, these have not been substantiated.

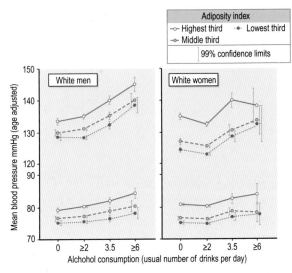

Fig. 3.3 Relationship between alcohol consumption and systolic and diastolic blood pressures, and the effect of body fat content. Blood pressure increases with increasing alcohol intake, and this effect is most marked in those with the highest adiposity indices. (From Klatsky et al © 1977,[16] Massachusetts Medical Society. All rights reserved.)

The hypertensive effects of alcohol are enhanced by increasing age, cigarette smoking and obesity (Fig. 3.3).[16] Moreover, regular alcohol consumption can also increase the requirements for anti-hypertensive medication. In the Atherosclerosis Risk in the Community study, it was estimated that in individuals who drank over 30 g alcohol per day (1 unit alcohol = 14 g alcohol), one in five cases of hypertension could be attributed to alcohol consumption.

PATTERN OF DRINKING

A large, population-based study of 1641 men in Finland showed that binge drinking is associated with increased morbidity and fatal myocardial infarction; this association is unrelated to the amount of alcohol consumed.

The mechanisms whereby alcohol consumption leads to raised blood pressure are unclear. There is some evidence to support the involvement of the sympathetic nervous system, endothelial

---

Box 3.9 Mechanisms of alcohol-associated hypertension

Stimulation of sympathetic nervous system
Stimulation of renin–angiotensin system
Increased insulin resistance
Endothelial dysfunction
Calcium and magnesium depletion

---

dysfunction, and depletion of electrolytes such as calcium and magnesium (Box 3.9).

ALCOHOL RESTRICTION AND BLOOD PRESSURE

Fifteen randomized controlled trials have examined the effect of decreased alcohol intake on blood pressure. Meta-analyses of these trials, which included 2235 individuals, showed the following.

- Alcohol restriction is associated with a 3-mmHg reduction in systolic blood pressure and a 2-mmHg reduction in diastolic blood pressure (Fig. 3.4).[17]

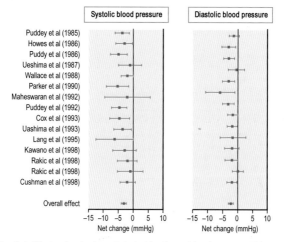

Fig. 3.4 Effects of reduction of alcohol intake on blood pressure. This meta-analysis showed that alcohol restriction is associated with average reductions of 3 and 2 mmHg in systolic and diastolic blood pressure, respectively. (From Xin et al 2001,[17] with permission of Lippincott, Williams and Wilkins.)

> **Box 3.10 Possible mechanisms involved in CHD risk reduction by alcohol**
>
> Increased HDL cholesterol
> Increased apolipoprotein A_1 and A_2
> Anti-oxidant effects
> Decreased fibrinogen
> Decreased platelet aggregation

- There is a clear dose–response relationship between the percentage alcohol reduction and mean blood pressure.
- Subjects with the highest baseline blood pressure achieve the greatest reductions in blood pressure following alcohol restriction.

ALCOHOL AND CHD

Paradoxically, regular drinking of between three and five standard drinks per day is associated with a reduced risk of CHD, despite increasing the risk of hypertension threefold. The beneficial effects of alcohol on CHD may be due to a number of effects (Box 3.10).

The absolute benefits of alcohol in terms of reduced CHD risk are likely to be greatest in those individuals at highest baseline risk. In practice, the benefits of reduced CHD risk associated with moderate drinking need to be balanced against the risks of hypertension, cardiomyopathy, arrhythmias and haemorrhagic stroke.

SMOKING

SMOKING AND BLOOD PRESSURE

Smoking is probably the most important modifiable risk factor for CHD[18] and premature death. In the UK, smoking accounts for 20% of CHD deaths in men and 17% in women. The NHS spends approximately £1500 million a year on the treatment of smoking-related diseases.

Interestingly, population-based studies show that chronic smoking tends to be associated with lower blood pressure, and that the prevalence of hypertension is lower in smokers. This association is probably explained by the fact that smokers have lower BMI values than non-smokers.

Acute smoking, however, is associated with a pressor effect, with a blood pressure increase of around 10/7 mmHg reported in hypertensive individuals 15 minutes after smoking two cigarettes. The pressor effect of acute smoking is potentiated by concomitant coffee drinking, both in terms of magnitude and duration. Using 24-hour ABPM, smokers with mild hypertension have been shown to have greater daytime blood pressure than those of non-smokers, despite the fact that blood pressure measured in the clinic is lower in the smokers.[19]

Hypertension is more difficult to control in smokers.

- Non-selective β blockers are less effective in smokers, probably due to vasoconstriction induced by unopposed α_1-receptor stimulation due to the rise in catecholamines associated with smoking.
- Hypertensive patients who smoke also have an increased risk of developing both renovascular and accelerated hypertension.

SMOKING AND CHD

- There is considerable evidence from randomized observational studies that smoking increases the risks of CHD and stroke, and that the risk is directly related to the number of cigarettes smoked.
- Although the risks for CHD may be less in cigar smokers, these risks should not be underestimated. A 1999 study of 17 774 men found that, compared with non-smokers, cigar smokers have an increased risk of CHD of 30%.[20]
- A 1999 meta-analysis has demonstrated that passive smoking is associated with an increase of 25% in the risk of CHD.[18]

SMOKING CESSATION AND CHD

Smoking cessation has been estimated to reduce the prevalence of CHD by around 43%.

Important: The benefits of smoking cessation occur rapidly: reductions in morbidity and mortality from CHD appear within 2 years.[21]

CAFFEINE

The reported effects of caffeine on blood pressure are inconsistent. Caffeine-containing drinks:

- increase blood pressure acutely
- produce an exaggerated response in patients with hypertension.

The majority of studies examining the long-term effects of caffeine on blood pressure have mostly studied coffee or tea and show no overall effect of long-term caffeine consumption on blood pressure. However, many of these studies excluded the elderly and patients with known hypertension.

Caffeine intake has been shown to potentiate the effects of smoking on blood pressure (see p. 109), and the combination of smoking and drinking caffeine-containing drinks should be avoided in patients with hypertension.

STRESS

Stress is an important environmental factor that may contribute to both the acute and chronic elevation of blood pressure. However, the role of stress in the genesis and long-term regulation of blood pressure is unclear, despite widespread public belief that they are intimately related.

The pressor effect of acute stress is well documented and undisputed. However, a number of strands of evidence suggest a link between stress and blood pressure in humans.

- Individuals of low socio-economic status living in 'high-stress' environments have higher blood pressure than similar individuals in 'low-stress' environments.
- Individuals with stressful jobs over which they have little control have higher average blood pressure levels than those with some degree of control. In addition, such individuals have an increased incidence of anxiety and depression.

It has also been suggested that individuals who suppress hostile emotions are more prone to develop hypertension. However, there are no randomized, controlled trials demonstrating that stress reduction techniques lower blood pressure.

FISH OIL

FISH OIL AND BLOOD PRESSURE

A number of trials have demonstrated that fish oil supplementation can reduce blood pressure. A systematic review looked at seven randomized controlled trials involving 339 individuals with hypertension.[22] The participants were mostly white, with an average

age of 50 years. The trials compared the effects of fish oil (mainly 3 g/day) versus no supplementation or placebo. However, the contents of the placebo capsules varied between trials. In addition, some fish oil mixtures contained omega-3 polyunsaturated fatty acids and some did not.

In comparison with control interventions, fish oil reduced systolic blood pressure by 4.5 mmHg and diastolic blood pressure by 2.5 mmHg. However, side effects were common and occurred in approximately a third of patients taking high-dose fish oil. Side effects included belching, bad breath, fishy taste and abdominal pain and diarrhoea.

FISH OIL AND CHD

There are no randomized controlled trials that have examined the effect of fish oil supplementation on morbidity and mortality in hypertensive patients. However, the following evidence is available.

- A number of randomized controlled trials have demonstrated that eating more fish oil or taking omega-3 polyunsaturated fatty acid supplementation improves survival in patients post myocardial infarction.[23,24]
- A meta-analysis of 11 randomized controlled trials (6–46 months' duration) of omega-3 polyunsaturated fatty acid supplementation (nine trials) or increased fish intake (two trials) demonstrated significant reduction in all-cause mortality, fatal myocardial infarction and sudden death, but not non-fatal myocardial infarction.[25]

The mechanisms of benefit from omega-3 polyunsaturated fatty acids are unclear but may be multiple (Box 3.11).

Box 3.11 Benefits of omega-3 polyunsaturated fatty acids

Decreased blood pressure
Improved endothelial function
Increased HDL cholesterol
Decreased platelet aggregation
Anti-arrhythmic effects
Anti-inflammatory effects
Decreased arterial stiffness

DIET

Links between blood pressure and diet have long been recognized
from data from population studies. Studies in vegetarians, both
population-based and clinical trials, consistently show lower blood
pressure in these individuals. However, no single dietary component
responsible has been identified.

DIET AND BLOOD PRESSURE

The DASH study investigated the effects on blood pressure of dietary
patterns previously reported to be associated with lower blood
pressure.[26]

REFERENCES

1. Cutler JA, Follmann D, Elliott P, et al. An overview of randomized trials
   of sodium reduction and blood pressure. Hypertension 1991; 17(1 Suppl):
   I27–I33.
2. Elliott P, Marmot M, Dyer A, et al. The INTERSALT study: main results,
   conclusions and some implications. Clin Exp Hypertens A 1989; 11(5–6):
   1025–1034.
3. Cutler JA, Follmann D, Allender PS. Randomized trials of
   sodium reduction: an overview. Am J Clin Nutr 1997; 65(2 Suppl):
   643S–651S.
4. Chobanian AV, Hill M. National Heart, Lung, and Blood Institute
   Workshop on Sodium and Blood Pressure: a critical review of current
   scientific evidence. Hypertension 2000; 35(4): 858–863.
5. Whelton PK, Appel LJ, Espeland MA, et al. Sodium reduction and weight
   loss in the treatment of hypertension in older persons: a randomized
   controlled trial of nonpharmacologic interventions in the elderly (TONE).
   TONE Collaborative Research Group. JAMA 1998; 279(11): 839–846.
6. Sacks FM, Svetkey LP, Vollmer WM, et al. Effects on blood pressure of
   reduced dietary sodium and the Dietary Approaches to Stop Hypertension
   (DASH) diet. DASH–Sodium Collaborative Research Group. N Engl J
   Med 2001; 344(1): 3–10.
7. Tuomilehto J, Jousilahti P, Rastenyte D, et al. Urinary sodium excretion
   and cardiovascular mortality in Finland: a prospective study. Lancet 2001;
   357(9259): 848–851.
8. Hooper L, Bartlett C, Davey SG, et al. Systematic review of long term
   effects of advice to reduce dietary salt in adults. Br Med J 2002;
   325(7365): 628.
9. Stamler R, Stamler J, Riedlinger WF, et al. Weight and blood pressure.
   Findings in hypertension screening of 1 million Americans. JAMA 1978;
   240(15): 1607–1610.

10. The Trials of Hypertension Prevention Collaborative Research Group. Effects of weight loss and sodium reduction intervention on blood pressure and hypertension incidence in overweight people with high-normal blood pressure. The Trials of Hypertension Prevention, phase II. Arch Intern Med 1997; 157(6): 657–667.

11. Blumenthal JA, Sherwood A, Gullette EC, et al. Exercise and weight loss reduce blood pressure in men and women with mild hypertension: effects on cardiovascular, metabolic, and hemodynamic functioning. Arch Intern Med 2000; 160(13): 1947–1958.

12. Berlin JA, Colditz GA. A meta-analysis of physical activity in the prevention of coronary heart disease. Am J Epidemiol 1990; 132(4): 612–628.

13. Whelton SP, Chin A, Xin X, et al. Effect of aerobic exercise on blood pressure: a meta-analysis of randomized, controlled trials. Ann Intern Med 2002; 136(7): 493–503.

14. Hayashi T, Tsumura K, Suematsu C, et al. Walking to work and the risk for hypertension in men: the Osaka Health Survey. Ann Intern Med 1999; 131(1): 21–26.

15. Hakim AA, Curb JD, Petrovitch H, et al. Effects of walking on coronary heart disease in elderly men: the Honolulu Heart Program. Circulation 1999; 100(1): 9–13.

16. Klatsky AL, Friedman GD, Siegelaub AB, et al. Alcohol consumption and blood pressure Kaiser-Permanente Multiphasic Health Examination data. N Engl J Med 1977; 296(21): 1194–1200.

17. Xin X, He J, Frontini MG, et al. Effects of alcohol reduction on blood pressure: a meta-analysis of randomized controlled trials. Hypertension 2001; 38(5): 1112–1117.

18. He J, Vupputuri S, Allen K, et al. Passive smoking and the risk of coronary heart disease—a meta-analysis of epidemiologic studies. N Engl J Med 1999; 340(12): 920–926.

19. Narkiewicz K, Maraglino G, Biasion T, et al. Interactive effect of cigarettes and coffee on daytime systolic blood pressure in patients with mild essential hypertension. HARVEST Study Group (Italy). Hypertension Ambulatory Recording VEnetia STudy. J Hypertens 1995; 13(9): 965–970.

20. Iribarren C, Tekawa IS, Sidney S, et al. Effect of cigar smoking on the risk of cardiovascular disease, chronic obstructive pulmonary disease, and cancer in men. N Engl J Med 1999; 340(23): 1773–1780.

21. Kawachi I, Colditz GA, Stampfer MJ, et al. Smoking cessation and time course of decreased risks of coronary heart disease in middle-aged women. Arch Intern Med 1994; 154(2): 169–175.

22. Morris MC, Sacks F, Rosner B. Does fish oil lower blood pressure? A meta-analysis of controlled trials. Circulation 1993; 88(2): 523–533.

23. Burr ML, Fehily AM, Gilbert JF, et al. Effects of changes in fat, fish, and fibre intakes on death and myocardial reinfarction: diet and reinfarction trial (DART). Lancet 1989; 2(8666): 757–761.

24. Gruppo Italiano per lo Studio della Sopravvivenza nell'Infarto miocardico. Dietary supplementation with n-3 polyunsaturated fatty acids and vitamin E

after myocardial infarction: results of the GISSI-Prevenzione trial. Lancet 1999; 354(9177): 447–455.

25. Marckmann P, Gronbaek M. Fish consumption and coronary heart disease mortality. A systematic review of prospective cohort studies. Eur J Clin Nutr 1999; 53(8): 585–590.

26. Appel LJ, Moore TJ, Obarzanek E, et al. A clinical trial of the effects of dietary patterns on blood pressure. DASH Collaborative Research Group. N Engl J Med 1997; 336(16): 1117–1124.

DRUG THERAPY FOR ESSENTIAL HYPERTENSION

PRINCIPLES OF THERAPY

The major objective of treating essential hypertension is to reduce cardiovascular morbidity and mortality while minimizing drug-related side-effects and maintaining the quality of life. Most clinicians would now accept that, for the majority of people, treatment should be based on total cardiovascular risk thresholds rather than the level of blood pressure alone.

- Aggressive management of other cardiovascular risk factors, such as hyperlipidaemia and diabetes, should be part of all treatment regimens for patients with essential hypertension.
- In addition, all patients should be actively advised on lifestyle modification (see *Lifestyle measures*, p. 97).

The majority of evidence suggests a continuous relationship between blood pressure and cardiovascular risk, with no threshold.[1] Therefore, in general, the lower the blood pressure the better.

BENEFITS BEYOND BLOOD PRESSURE REDUCTION

The past decade has seen intense debate and controversy as to whether the benefit of lowering blood pressure in terms of cardiovascular outcome is due to blood pressure reduction *per se*, or whether the class of anti-hypertensive agent used provides additional benefit.

Despite early belief that the newer anti-hypertensive agents such as calcium channel blockers, angiotensin-converting enzyme (ACE) inhibitors, and most recently angiotensin II receptor blockers may affect prognosis beyond their effects on blood pressure alone, this has not been substantiated in practice. For example, the Antihypertensive and Lipid-Lowering Treatment to Prevent Heart Attack Trial (ALLHAT) showed no difference in outcome between patients treated with regimens based on calcium channel blocker, thiazide diuretic and ACE inhibitor.[2]

The only exception to this pattern may be observed in comparisons with traditional β blockers such as atenolol. The Losartan Intervention for Endpoint Reduction in Hypertension (LIFE) study suggested that an anti-hypertensive regimen based on atenolol reduces cardiovascular events (mostly stroke) less than one based on an angiotensin II receptor antagonist for the same degree of blood pressure reduction.[3] This effect may be due to the relatively poor effects that β blockers have on reducing central aortic blood pressure. Interestingly, β blockers were also inferior to thiazide diuretics in the

MRC Elderly Study. A recent meta-analysis in the *Lancet* has questioned the efficacy of atenolol, in particular, in reducing mortality in hypertensive patients.[14] However, whether other β blockers are better in this respect remains to be established, although vasodilating β blockers do appear to have some physiological advantage.

Despite the above, the overall message from a number of meta-analyses of the major hypertension trials, including the LIFE study, is that there has been a failure to demonstrate benefit from any class of anti-hypertensive agent beyond blood pressure reduction alone.[4–6]

IMPORTANCE OF BLOOD PRESSURE CONTROL

The findings described—that differences in blood pressure largely account for cardiovascular outcome—emphasize the desirability of tight blood pressure control. Despite this, essential hypertension remains under-diagnosed and under-treated, resulting in significant numbers of strokes and heart attacks that are potentially preventable. Indeed, even in patients with hypertension and established coronary heart disease, blood pressure is insufficiently controlled.[7] Furthermore, implementation of hypertension management guidelines has considerable cost implications,[8] especially in less developed countries.

THIAZIDE DIURETICS

Thiazide diuretics are inexpensive and have the most evidence for efficacy. The largest hypertension trial to date, ALLHAT, showed that treatment with a diuretic is equally as effective as either an ACE inhibitor or a calcium channel blocker (Fig. 3.5).[2] Indeed, a 2003 systematic review of meta-analyses and journal reviews suggested that, in patients with essential hypertension, low-dose diuretics are as effective as or more effective than other anti-hypertensive agents as first-line therapy in preventing major cardiovascular end points.[9] Thiazide diuretics may therefore be the preferred first-line anti-hypertensive for the majority of hypertensive patients, as was recommended in the recent NICE guidance[15] (see p. 119) on the management of hypertension.

THE ABCD RULE

In the 2004 British Hypertension Society guidelines, the ABCD rule is used to guide the choice of drug therapy for patients with hypertension (Fig. 3.6).[10] This rule is based on the following facts.

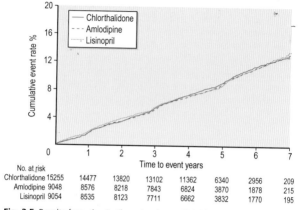

Fig. 3.5 Results from the Antihypertensive and Lipid-Lowering Treatment to Prevent Heart Attack Trial. No significant difference in the primary outcome (fatal coronary heart disease or non-fatal myocardial infarction) was seen between the patient groups treated with chlorthalidone, amlodipine or lisinopril. (From ALLHAT 2002,[2] with permission.)

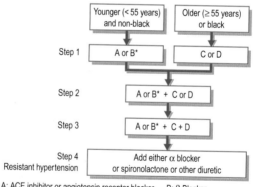

A: ACE inhibitor or angiotensin receptor blocker   B: β Blocker
C: Calcium channel blocker
D: Diuretic (thiazide and thiazide-like)

* Combination therapy involving B and D may induce more new-onset diabetes compared with other combination therapies

Fig. 3.6 Adapted from the ABCD rule for choice of anti-hypertensive therapy: a stepwise approach to the drug therapy for hypertension. (From Williams 2004,[10] with permission.)

> **Box 3.12 Hypertensive target organ damage**
>
> Myocardial infarction
> Stroke
> Angina
> Heart failure
> Transient ischaemic attack
> Chronic renal failure
> Peripheral vascular disease

- Younger patients, who usually have relatively high renin levels, are likely to respond better to drugs acting on the renin–angiotensin system, such as ACE inhibitors, angiotensin receptor antagonists or β blockers (A or B).
- Older patients, with relatively low renin levels, are likely to respond better to calcium channel blockers or thiazide diuretics (C or D).

Therefore the first-line choice of drug is guided by the patient's age.

If combination therapy is necessary, the ABCD rule also guides the best initial approach to combining drugs. In general, drugs from the two different groups are used together, such that they act in a complementary fashion against the compensatory physiological effects produced by the other group of drugs (i.e. if two drugs are to be used, A or B should be combined with C or D). High-risk individuals with systolic blood pressure greater than 160 mmHg or with diabetes or target organ damage (Box 3.12) should be treated with two or more drugs.

The recent NICE guidance[15] on the management of hypertension suggests an alternative approach, with all patients starting on a thiazide diuretic, unless contra-indicated. If the diuretic is not tolerated or is ineffective a β blocker is substituted. Once combination therapy is required, a similar approach to the ABCD rule is followed.

Although the NICE and British Hypertension Society guidelines appear to be at variance, since most patients with hypertension are aged over 60, the majority will be started on a thiazide first-line whichever algorithm is followed.

IDEAL BLOOD PRESSURE REDUCTION

Despite overwhelming evidence as to the benefits of blood pressure reduction in terms of preventing cardiovascular events, the level to which blood pressure must be reduced to achieve maximum benefit remains unknown.

TARGETS OF THERAPY

A number of evidence-based guidelines have been produced in which blood pressure targets have been identified. These include:

- the American Joint National Committee guidelines (JNC 7)[11]
- the joint European Society of Hypertension and European Society of Cardiology guidelines.[12]

Both sets of guidelines emphasize the importance of treating all cardiovascular risk factors, and as such set lower blood pressure targets for patients with hypertension at highest cardiovascular risk, especially those with diabetes and chronic renal failure (Fig. 3.7).

The American guidelines, JNC 7, have for the first time introduced the concept of pre-hypertension (systolic blood pressure 130–139 mmHg and diastolic pressure 80–89 mmHg). Although there is no recommendation for drug treatment in patients in this group, they should receive lifestyle modification if necessary.

Although blood pressure targets will change with evidence provided from ongoing blood pressure trials, it would appear that the lower the blood pressure the better, especially in patients with additional cardiovascular risk factors.

Finally, the increasing incidence of isolated systolic hypertension (a disease associated with vascular ageing) means that in longer-lived societies the incidence of hypertension will increase dramatically. Indeed, JNC 7 states that the evidence is that an individual who is normotensive at age 55 has a lifetime risk of developing hypertension of 90%.

COMPLIANCE

> **Important:** The evidence from the hypertension trials demonstrates beyond doubt that patients with essential hypertension will benefit from blood pressure reduction, and that the greater the blood pressure reduction the greater the benefit, irrespective of the anti-hypertensive agent used.

The extent to which patients comply with recommended therapies is known as compliance (or concordance). Compliance is a major issue in the control of blood pressure and depends on a number of factors (Box 3.13). As target blood pressures have fallen—and hence

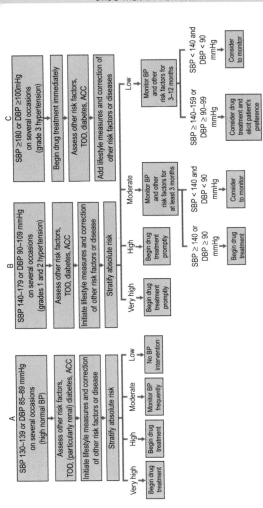

Fig. 3.7 European Society of Hypertension–European Society of Cardiology guidelines for the management of arterial hypertension: algorithm for initiating anti-hypertensive treatment based on initial blood pressure levels (A, B or C) and total risk level. SBP, systolic blood pressure; DBP, diastolic blood pressure; BP, blood pressure; TOD, target organ damage; ACC, associated clinical conditions. (After Guidelines Committee 2003,¹² with permission of Lippincott, Williams and Wilkins.)

Box 3.13 Factors affecting compliance with anti-hypertensive therapy and lifestyle advice

Factors that improve compliance
Regular visits to the doctor
Other coexisting illnesses
Desire to control blood pressure
Fear of complications of hypertension
Simple medication regimen
Home blood pressure monitoring
Family support
Health insurance

Factors that worsen compliance
Non-healthy behaviour such as smoking, excess alcohol intake and sedentary lifestyle
Social factors
Patient belief systems
Concern about side effects of medications
Complicated multiple drug regimen
Cost

the number of drugs given to patients both to control their blood pressure and to reduce other cardiovascular risk factors has increased—compliance has become an even bigger problem.

Strategies to improve compliance fall into three major categories: actions by patients, actions by health care providers, and actions by health care organizations.

Actions that fall into the first of these categories are as follows.

- Patients need to control all risk factors and should negotiate and agree sensible attainable goals with their doctor or nurse.
- They should be encouraged to develop skills to maintain recommended behaviour patterns.
- Monitoring of progress towards agreed goals is also important, and problems blocking attainment of the goals should be resolved in partnership with the doctor.

For their part, doctors and nurses should do the following.

- Provide clear, direct, easily understandable messages about the importance of a particular behaviour or therapeutic intervention. To this end, patients should be involved in therapeutic decisions.

- Document progress towards agreed goals and provide patients with feedback on their progress.
- Patient compliance should be assessed at each clinic visit.

At the organizational level, several approaches can improve compliance.

- Health care organizations should foster and support environments that emphasize prevention and treatment interventions.
- They should provide high-quality tracking and reporting systems.
- They should provide evidence-based updates and training for doctors and nurses treating hypertension and rapidly incorporate any innovations into clinical practice.

In the future, developments such as telemedicine and virtual hypertension clinics may improve both patients' recording of their own blood pressure and adherence to therapy.

ASSESSING RESPONSE TO THERAPY

Despite the provision of clear, comprehensive, evidence-based guidelines for the management of hypertension, clinical management often fails to achieve the evidence-based targets for adequate blood pressure control or the optimal choice of anti-hypertensive agent.

PATIENT-HELD RECORDS

To manage hypertension optimally over time, doctors and other health care professionals need to constantly assess the response to therapy. To do this, they need rapid, accurate access to the patients' medical records in terms of previous blood pressure readings and anti-hypertensive regimens. Such information has been traditionally difficult for doctors to extract from clinic charts. Indeed, information in traditional clinic notes can be so extensive that it overwhelms the doctor's ability to evaluate it effectively in the time available for a clinic or general practitioner consultation, and as such presents a barrier to blood pressure control.

The advent of patient-held records on which current medication and evidence-based blood pressure targets are clearly stated has improved the situation. Presentation of data in a graphic form can further improve both the patient's and the doctor's perception of important patterns. In the future, advances in technology will allow for patient-held electronic records, which will improve the assessment of response to therapy still more.

A ROLE FOR TELEMEDICINE

The next few years are likely to see increased use of telemedicine systems, whereby a patient can take repeated home blood pressure readings (or 24-hour readings) and download the data over the telephone line. This allows the doctor access to accurate home-based data on which to assess the patient's response to therapy, thus creating a virtual hypertension clinic. Such schemes are already showing promise in terms of improving follow-up and assessment to treatment.

FOLLOW-UP INTERVALS

Interestingly, a 2004 study involving 609 subjects with hypertension compared 3- versus 6-month follow-up periods in general practice.[13] Patient satisfaction and adherence to therapy was the same, irrespective of follow-up intervals. Hypertension in approximately 20% of patients was uncontrolled at any time in either group, suggesting that frequency of follow-up is unlikely to be the most important factor in terms of assessment of response to therapy in general practice.

REFERENCES

1. Lewington S, Clarke R, Qizilbash N, et al. Age-specific relevance of usual blood pressure to vascular mortality: a meta-analysis of individual data for one million adults in 61 prospective studies. Lancet 2002; 360(9349): 1903–1913.
2. ALLHAT Officers and Coordinators. Major outcomes in high-risk hypertensive patients randomized to angiotensin-converting enzyme inhibitor or calcium channel blocker vs diuretic: the Antihypertensive and Lipid-Lowering Treatment to Prevent Heart Attack Trial (ALLHAT). JAMA 2002; 288(23): 2981–2997.
3. Dahlof B, Devereux RB, Kjeldsen SE, et al. Cardiovascular morbidity and mortality in the Losartan Intervention For Endpoint reduction in hypertension study (LIFE): a randomised trial against atenolol. Lancet 2002; 359(9311): 995–1003.
4. Staessen JA, Wang JG, Thijs L. Cardiovascular protection and blood pressure reduction: a meta-analysis. Lancet 2001; 358(9290): 1305–1315.
5. Staessen JA, Wang JG, Thijs L. Cardiovascular prevention and blood pressure reduction: a quantitative overview updated until 1 March 2003. J Hypertens 2003; 21(6): 1055–1076.
6. Turnbull F. Effects of different blood-pressure–lowering regimens on major cardiovascular events: results of prospectively designed overviews of randomised trials. Lancet 2003; 362(9395): 1527–1535.

7. Boersma E, Keil U, De Bacquer D, et al. Blood pressure is insufficiently controlled in European patients with established coronary heart disease. J Hypertens 2003; 21(10): 1831–1840.

8. Zanchetti A. Costs of implementing recommendations on hypertension management given in recent guidelines. J Hypertens 2003; 21(12): 2207–2209.

9. Psaty BM, Lumley T, Furberg CD, et al. Health outcomes associated with various antihypertensive therapies used as first-line agents: a network meta-analysis. JAMA 2003; 289(19): 2534–2544.

10. Williams B, Poulter NR, Brown MJ, et al. Guidelines for management of hypertension: report of the fourth working party of the British Hypertension Society, 2004—BHS IV. J Hum Hypertens 2004; 18(3): 139–185.

11. Chobanian AV, Bakris GL, Black HR, et al. The seventh report of the Joint National Committee on Prevention, Detection, Evaluation, and Treatment of High Blood Pressure: the JNC 7 report. JAMA 2003; 289(19): 2560–2572.

12. Guidelines Committee 2003 European Society of Hypertension–European Society of Cardiology guidelines for the management of arterial hypertension. J Hypertens 2003; 21(6): 1011–1053.

13. Birtwhistle RV, Godwin MS, Delva MD, et al. Randomised equivalence trial comparing three month and six month follow up of patients with hypertension by family practitioners. Br Med J 2004; 328(7433): 204.

14. Carlberg B, Samuelsson O, Lindholm LH. Atenolol in hypertension: is it a wise choice? Lancet 2004; 364(9446): 1684–1689.

15. NICE Guideline. CG18 Hypertension (persistently high blood pressure) in adults. 2004. www.nice.org.uk/pdf/word/CGO18NICEguidelineword.doc

MAJOR DRUG CLASSES IN HYPERTENSION

THIAZIDE DIURETICS

Thiazide diuretics, when they were introduced to clinical practice in the 1950s, were the first effective, well-tolerated, oral anti-hypertensive agents and they revolutionized the management of hypertension. Thiazide diuretics are ideal first-line agents in the treatment of hypertension because they produce a predictable sustained reduction in blood pressure in at least 50% of patients, with no serious adverse effects. In addition, over the past 50 years numerous trials have proved that thiazide diuretics reduce cardiovascular morbidity and mortality in both systolic and diastolic hypertension.

MECHANISM OF ACTION

The anti-hypertensive effects of thiazide diuretics can be divided into three phases.

- Acute phase (1–2 weeks). During this phase, thiazides act by inhibiting the sodium chloride pump in the distal convoluted tubule, which leads to increased urinary sodium excretion. Initially this results in a variable reduction in the extracellular fluid volume, a fall in cardiac output, and a compensatory rise in peripheral vascular resistance. However, blood volume returns to normal within a few days of starting therapy.
- Sub-acute phase (4–8 weeks). During this phase, cardiac output and peripheral resistance are both lower.
- Chronic phase (2–3 months). During this phase, the system 'resets' due to counter-regulatory mechanisms, and cardiac output and peripheral resistance return to normal, but blood pressure remains lowered. The exact cellular mechanism for this relative vasodilatation remains unclear but most probably involves alteration in vascular cell ion transport.[1]

ADVERSE EFFECTS

When first introduced into clinical practice at high doses (up to 200 mg/day of hydrochlorothiazide), metabolic side effects of diuretics were used to explain the failure of these drugs to produce the expected reduction in myocardial infarction in the early large hypertension studies. However, since then several other studies using different agents have shown that, in most cases, anti-hypertensive therapy tends to reduce stroke risk more than myocardial infarction risk; therefore this finding is not confined to thiazide diuretics. Moreover, lower doses of thiazides are now employed (e.g. 12.5–25 mg hydrochlorothiazide), and these are as effective as higher doses in terms of blood pressure control but are usually metabolically neutral.

Overall, thiazides probably have the largest body of evidence demonstrating benefit of any anti-hypertensive drugs, and they significantly reduce cardiovascular risk, especially in the elderly, rendering the initial concerns as to the safety of thiazides unfounded.

Hyponatraemia

This side effect is uncommon, especially in patients treated with low doses. However, rarely, diuretic-induced hyponatraemia may occur as an idiosyncratic reaction in patients on low-dose therapy. This can be rapidly corrected by:

- discontinuation of the diuretic
- increased sodium intake
- water restriction (if necessary).

Hypokalaemia

Thiazide diuretics tend to cause a dose-related metabolic alkalosis, and less than 10% of patients develop mild hypokalaemia on low-dose thiazide therapy.

There has been much previous controversy as to thiazide-induced hypokalaemia and the risk of ventricular arrhythmias and sudden death suggested by the early blood pressure trials. This suggested association has not been confirmed in subsequent studies, and the Antihypertensive and Lipid-Lowering Treatment to Prevent Heart Attack Trial (ALLHAT) showed that small reductions in potassium do not increase the risk of sudden death.[2]

Thiazide-induced hypokalaemia may increase risk in patients with heart failure, especially if they are also treated with digoxin.

Lipids and glucose

Again, early trials suggested that thiazides cause adverse increases in lipids and glucose. However, currently recommended doses of thiazides have a negligible effect on serum lipids.

The diabetic potential of thiazides has also been a cause for concern, and some clinicians were wary of introducing thiazides to the regimen of patients with diabetes. However, the Systolic Hypertension in the Elderly Program (SHEP) study used a diuretic-based regimen and showed a significantly greater benefit in diabetic patients treated with a thiazide compared with that in the non-diabetic group.[3] In ALLHAT, the incidence of diabetes in the thiazide group was 12%, compared with 8% in patients on the angiotensin-converting enzyme (ACE) inhibitor lisinopril.

Gout
Thiazide-induced hyperuricaemia occurs as the result of volume contraction or due to competition of thiazides with uric acid for renal tubular secretion via the organic anion pathway. Therefore gouty arthritis can be precipitated in susceptible individuals, but this is uncommon.

Impotence
Impotence is a side effect of thiazides but is uncommon (occurring in less than 2%) on low doses and resolves on stopping the drug.

Hypomagnesaemia
Although reasonably common, the clinical significance of hypomagnesaemia is unclear. However, it may increase the tendency to hypokalaemia and cardiac arrhythmias, and make the correction of hypokalaemia difficult in a few patients.

β BLOCKERS

β Blockers are effective and safe, and they are widely used in the treatment of hypertension and other cardiovascular disorders. The pharmacological characteristics of β blockers are similar, in that they are competitive inhibitors of the effects of catecholamines at β-adrenergic receptors.

- The so-called 'cardio-selective' β blockers bind preferentially to the β_1 adrenoceptor. However, this selectivity is progressively lost with increasing dosage.
- Some β blockers, for example pindolol, have partial agonist activity that is intrinsic sympathomimetic activity. Such agents not only antagonize the effects of circulating catecholamines but also stimulate the β receptor; their overall effect will therefore be dependent on the dosage used.
- Other β blockers, such as labetalol, exhibit both β- and α-adrenoceptor antagonism, and as such exhibit some vasodilating activity.
- The β blocker sotalol has the additional effect of potassium channel blockade leading to class III anti-arrhythmic effects.
- The recently available β blocker nebivolol has been shown to release nitric oxide from the vascular endothelium and produces vasodilatation in both normotensive and hypertensive individuals.

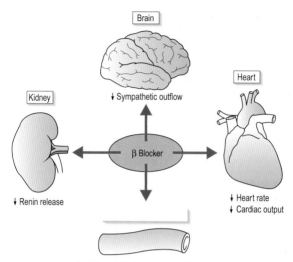

Fig. 3.8 Potential mechanism of action of β blockers. The initial vasoconstriction of peripheral blood vessels produced by β blockade would tend to increase peripheral resistance and blood pressure, but this effect is offset by a decreased heart rate and cardiac output. Unlike the other β blockers, the newer β blocker nebivolol produces vasodilatation in the peripheral vascular bed via nitric oxide release. NO, nitric oxide. (From Cockcroft 1999,[4] with permission of Prescriber.)

When given acutely, non-selective β blockers increase peripheral vascular resistance, but this effect is offset by a concomitant decrease in heart rate and cardiac output, and the acute effect on blood pressure is therefore neutral. However, significant reductions in blood pressure are obtained with chronic β-blocker therapy, the exact mechanisms of which remain unclear but may well involve resetting of baroreceptors. Other possible mechanisms involved in the anti-hypertensive effect of β blockers are shown in Fig. 3.8 and Box 3.14.

INDICATIONS FOR THE USE OF β BLOCKERS

β Blockers have been used for several years in the treatment of hypertension, and their efficacy in terms of lowering blood pressure has been demonstrated in many studies.[5–7] However, in terms of outcome, the overall data suggest that β blockers may be less

> **Box 3.14 Mechanisms involved in the anti-hypertensive effects of β blockers**
>
> Reduction in heart rate and cardiac output
> Decreases in central sympathetic outflow
> Decreased renin release from the kidney (because this is sympathetically mediated)
> Reduction in peripheral vascular resistance, especially in drugs with intrinsic sympathomimetic activity, those with α-blocking activity, and nebivolol (which releases NO)
> Resetting of baroreceptor function
> Inhibition of pre-junctional β receptors to decrease noradrenaline release
> Attenuation of the pressor response to exercise and stress

effective than other anti-hypertensive agents in reducing cardiovascular risk, especially in older patients with hypertension, and particularly in isolated systolic hypertension.[8]

The MRC trial of treatment of hypertension in older adults compared treatment with atenolol, hydrochlorothiazide or amiloride, and placebo. The researchers concluded that—despite an overall reduction in stroke, coronary events and all-cardiovascular events in the treatment group compared with the placebo group—when looked at alone, the β-blocker group showed no significant reduction in these end points.[9] Indeed, one systematic review of trials using β blockers in the elderly concluded that diuretic therapy is superior to β blockade with regard to all end points.[10]

The Losartan Intervention for Endpoint Reduction in Hypertension (LIFE) study compared the β blocker atenolol with the angiotensin II receptor blocker losartan in older hypertensive patients (Fig. 3.9).[11] Despite similar degrees of blood pressure reduction, more cardiovascular events were prevented in the losartan-treated group, the major contribution being a reduction in stroke. However, blood pressure was measured peripherally using conventional sphygmomanometry, and because β blockade may augment central aortic pressure (which is the pressure the heart actually sees), there may have been a significant difference in aortic pressure between the two treatment groups. Further studies will be needed that include non-invasive measurement of central aortic pressure to resolve this issue.

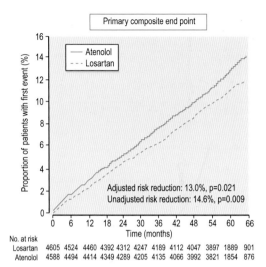

Fig. 3.9 The Losartan Intervention for Endpoint Reduction in Hypertension (LIFE) study. In hypertensive patients with left ventricular hypertrophy, there was a reduction in the risk of cardiovascular morbidity and mortality in patients treated with a losartan-based anti-hypertensive regimen compared with those treated with an atenolol-based regimen. (From Dahlof et al 2002,[11] with permission from Elsevier.)

Despite the above results, β blockers are useful drugs in lowering blood pressure.

- β Blockers are particularly effective in younger patients, who tend to have higher renin levels and increased cardiac output in the initial phase of hypertension; first-line therapy with β blockers may be appropriate in these patients.
- They may be the first-line choice for patients with hypertension combined with angina or certain cardiac arrhythmias.
- β Blockers may be preferred following myocardial infarction, because they reduce sudden death and re-infarction rates.

Important: β Blockers are *not* usually used as first-line treatment in black patients, because this group of patients tends to respond better to other classes of drug (such as the diuretics or calcium channel blockers).

Because the majority of hypertensive patients will require more than one drug to achieve blood pressure targets, β blockers also have a major role in combination therapy; for example, the combination of β blockers with calcium channel blockers (except verapamil) is a well-established and effective therapeutic approach.

TOLERABILITY

β Blockers are well tolerated by the majority of patients. However, side effects can occur, especially in individuals treated with high doses of β blockers.

> **Important:** Side effects tend to be less common for the less lipid-soluble β blockers (such as atenolol), because they are less likely to cross the blood–brain barrier.

Central side-effects of β blockers include:

- tiredness
- nightmares
- insomnia
- vivid dreams.

Although some small studies have suggested that depression is associated with β blockade, this suggestion has not been supported in a meta-analysis.[12] Although erectile dysfunction was a side effect of β blockade in the MRC blood pressure trial, this side effect was equally common in patients taking thiazide diuretics.

> **Important:** Side-effects of β blockers include cold extremities, and these drugs (except perhaps nebivolol) should be avoided in patients with Raynaud's disease or severe peripheral vascular disease. β Blockers are contra-indicated in patients with asthma and in some patients with chronic obstructive pulmonary disease because they cause bronchoconstriction.

CALCIUM CHANNEL BLOCKERS

Calcium channel blockers are powerful arterial dilators, and as such are useful as mono-therapy or in combination with other anti-

TABLE 3.1 Classes of calcium channel blockers

	Dihydropyridines	Non-dihydropyridines	
		Phenylalkylamines	Benzothiazepines
Examples	Nifedipine, amlodipine, lercanidipine	Verapamil	Diltiazem
Effect on heart rate	Increase	Decrease	Decrease
Site of action	Vasculature	Vasculature and heart	Vasculature and heart
Side effects	Headache, ankle swelling (less with lercanidipine), flushing	Constipation, heart failure, heart block	Heart failure, heart block, constipation

hypertensive agents. Data suggest that they are particularly useful in the prevention of stroke.

Calcium channel blockers are a structurally and pharmacologically diverse group of agents that can be divided into three major categories:

- 1,4-dihydropyridines
- phenylalkylamines
- benzothiazepines.

The latter two categories are classed as the non-dihydropyridines. The different classes of calcium channel blocker bind to different sites, thus giving them slightly different actions and side-effect profiles (Table 3.1). However, all of these agents reduce blood pressure by decreasing cellular calcium entry via the L-type calcium channel.

> **Important:** Dihydropyridine calcium channel blockers decrease blood pressure by reducing peripheral vascular resistance. Usually this is accompanied by a reflex tachycardia and sympathetic activation, which can be counteracted in clinical practice by combination with a β blocker.

The non-dihydropyridines also decrease peripheral vascular resistance, but in addition they decrease myocardial contractility and heart rate. This leads to a fall in cardiac output, which also contributes to their anti-hypertensive action.

> **Box 3.15 Indications for the use of calcium channel blockers in hypertension**
>
> Isolated systolic hypertension
> Black patients with hypertension
> Hypertensive patients on concomitant therapy with non-steroidal anti-inflammatory drugs
> Patients with isolated systolic hypertension and diabetes
> Patients with hypertension and unstable angina, especially those unable to tolerate β blockade
> Patients at high risk of developing type 2 diabetes
> Patients over 55 years of age
> Patients post-myocardial infarction (diltiazem and verapamil)
> Hypertension related to ciclosporin therapy

INDICATIONS FOR THE USE OF CALCIUM CHANNEL BLOCKERS

Box 3.15 lists indications for calcium channel blockers. In addition to their use in hypertension, calcium channel blockers are used in angina, and verapamil is useful in the treatment of some arrhythmias. Calcium channel blockers are generally effective and safe, with response rates to mono-therapy in hypertension of greater than 50%.

- Calcium channel blockers are equally effective in black and white patients, and unlike other anti-hypertensives their efficacy is maintained independent of salt intake or concomitant non-steroidal anti-inflammatory drug (NSAID) usage.
- They are also effective in patients with ciclosporin-induced hypertension. Indeed, nifedipine—which inhibits the metabolism of ciclosporin—is sometimes used in renal units to decrease the amount of ciclosporin used to prevent rejection; this has led to considerable cost reduction.

> **Important:** Calcium channel blockers are especially effective in isolated systolic hypertension, a common condition in the elderly that is characterized by increased large arterial stiffening manifest as a wide peripheral pulse pressure.

Two trials in patients with isolated systolic hypertension, Syst–Eur and Syst–China, have been based on treatment with a calcium channel blocker. In the Syst–Eur study, the dihydropyridine nitrendipine decreased stroke by 40%, and all-cause cardiovascular mortality and morbidity by 30%. The Hypertension Optimal Treatment (HOT) trial was based on a regimen using felodipine and demonstrated that decreasing blood pressure below 140/90 mmHg is safe and effective.

In the largest blood pressure study to date, ALLHAT, reduction of blood pressure by the calcium channel blocker amlodipine was approximately 4 mmHg greater than that achieved with the ACE inhibitor lisinopril and approximately 2 mmHg greater than the diuretic chlorthalidone, although cardiovascular outcome was similar for all three patient groups.

A large number of randomized trials have demonstrated that blood pressure reduction is particularly effective in reducing cardiovascular morbidity and mortality in subjects with type 2 diabetes. Indeed, because those with diabetes are at increased baseline risk of cardiovascular disease, the absolute reduction of risk with anti-hypertensive therapy is greater than that in non-diabetic individuals. This is supported by data from the Syst–Eur study, which was conducted in patients with isolated systolic hypertension and used a regimen based on the calcium channel blocker nitrendipine: subjects with diabetes achieved greater benefit from blood pressure reduction than those without diabetes.

> **Important:** Evidence has suggested that both thiazide diuretics and β blockers may increase the incidence of type 2 diabetes, especially when used in combination. Therefore calcium channel blockers may be useful in patients with hypertension and additional risk factors for diabetes, such as obesity and a strong family history of type 2 diabetes.

CONTRA-INDICATIONS TO THE USE OF CALCIUM CHANNEL BLOCKERS

Use in patients with renal disease

To date, clinical trials suggest that calcium channel blockade may not be as protective against the progression of renal disease as ACE inhibitors or angiotensin receptor blockers. However, the second phase of the Appropriate Blood Pressure Control in Diabetes (ABCD) study demonstrated that, in diabetic individuals with normal renal function, the calcium channel blocker nisoldipine is equally effective in protecting against deterioration in renal function. More evidence will therefore be necessary before renal impairment is considered an absolute contra-indication to the use of calcium channel blockade.

Use in patients with heart failure

Because many calcium channel blockers, especially the non-dihydropyridines, are negatively inotropic, their use in patients with heart failure has been subject to much debate.

A number of trials have examined the effect of calcium channel blockers in individuals with left ventricular dysfunction. In the Prospective Randomized Amlodipine Survival Evaluation (PRAISE) trial, amlodipine was found to be 'neutral', that is, relatively safe but not beneficial when added to the regimen of patients already taking diuretics and ACE inhibitors.[13] In ALLHAT, however, the calcium channel blocker amlodipine was inferior to the diuretic chlorthalidone in preventing heart failure.

> **Important:** Although calcium channel blockers are probably safe in patients with heart failure, they should be introduced with caution and should not generally be used in patients with significant risk of heart failure or those with overt clinical evidence of heart failure.

- The non-dihydropyridine calcium channel blocker verapamil, in addition to its negatively inotropic effect, produces partial blockade of both the atrioventricular (AV) and sinoatrial (SA) nodes; this drug should *not* therefore be used in combination with a β blocker.
- In patients with aortic stenosis or complete heart block, calcium channel blockers should only be used with caution and are probably best avoided.

Adverse effects

Adverse effects seen with calcium channel blockade will depend on the type of agent used (see Table 3.1). The dihydropyridines are associated with:

- flushing
- headaches
- postural dizziness
- palpitations
- tachycardia
- ankle oedema.

Ankle oedema can be especially problematic. It is not due to net salt and water retention caused by peripheral vasodilatation, but by a greater dilatation of the arteriolar rather than the venous circulation, giving rise to a raised trans-capillary gradient and capillary leakage.

> **Important:** ACE inhibitors may be effective in reducing ankle oedema associated with calcium channel blockade because they lower tissue hydrostatic pressure by a balanced arteriolar–venous dilatation.

Effects on cardiovascular outcome

The evidence-base for the use of calcium channel blockers has been discussed, in part, above, especially their efficacy in patients with isolated systolic hypertension. It has been expanded by two large studies, the International Nifedipine GITS Study: Intervention as a Goal in Hypertension Treatment (INSIGHT) (Fig. 3.10)[14] and the Nordic Diltiazem Study (NORDIL),[15] using the calcium channel blockers nifedipine gastrointestinal therapeutic system (GITS) and diltiazem, respectively. The studies were in agreement and demonstrated that both agents are equally effective at reducing cardiovascular outcome as regimens based on diuretics or β blockers.

> **Important:** Calcium channel blockers appear to be especially effective in preventing stroke; this was shown by a 2001 meta-analysis of nine randomized trials involving 62 605 patients (although blood pressure reduction *per se* is what produces most benefit).[16]

ACE INHIBITORS

The ACE inhibitors act by inhibiting the conversion of the inactive decapeptide angiotensin I to the active octapeptide angiotensin II, which is a powerful vasoconstrictor and acts via an increase in aldosterone production to retain salt and water.

When the first ACE inhibitor, captopril, was introduced into clinical practice, it was thought that it would not be a particularly effective anti-hypertensive agent, because the majority of patients with essential hypertension have low or normal renin levels and were, therefore, unlikely to have activated renin–angiotensin systems. However, when used clinically, ACE inhibitors rapidly establish

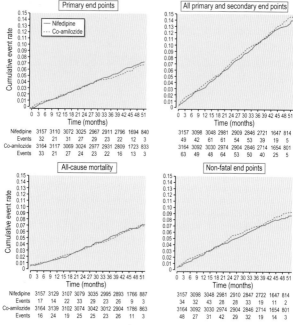

Fig. 3.10 The International Nifedipine GITS Study: Intervention as a Goal in Hypertension Treatment (INSIGHT). There was no significant difference in outcome between patients treated with a nifedipine-based anti-hypertensive regimen and those treated with a co-amilozide-based regimen. (From Brown et al 2000,[14] with permission from Elsevier.)

themselves as highly effective at lowering blood pressure across a broad spectrum of patients with hypertension, suggesting that they may act via mechanisms other than just inhibition of ACE. This is supported by the fact that the blood pressure fall produced by ACE inhibition is often unrelated to the circulating plasma renin activity.

- Because ACE also degrades the vasodilator peptide bradykinin, ACE inhibitors may act via potentiating circulating levels of bradykinin. Indeed, a study using the bradykinin receptor blocker HOE-140 has demonstrated that the hypotensive effect of ACE inhibition can be blunted by around 20% in patients given both compounds together.
- Angiotensin II also acts to produce indirect vasoconstriction by potentiation of the sympathetic nervous system via an increased

release of noradrenaline at pre-synaptic nerve terminals. Because angiotensin II can also potentiate the post-synaptic action of noradrenaline, ACE inhibitors will thus decrease sympathetic nervous system activity.

● Because bradykinin enhances the synthesis of a number of vasodilator prostanoids, ACE inhibition will increase their circulating levels, leading to further vasodilatation.

In hypertension, ACE inhibition produces a balanced reduction of both cardiac pre-load and after-load through direct and indirect arteriolar dilatation. The ACE inhibitors also blunt stress-induced increases in catecholamines via their sympatholytic effects, and thus heart rate changes with ACE inhibition are not significant.

It has been suggested that long-term ACE inhibition may be associated with the phenomenon of angiotensin II escape due to generation of angiotensin II by non-ACE-mediated pathways. Because ACE inhibitors will increase levels of angiotensin I by blocking its conversion to angiotensin II, the increased circulating levels of angiotensin I may provide a substrate for other enzymes (such as kinases) to generate angiotensin II. Such pathways would not be blocked by ACE inhibitors, and this led some researchers to speculate that complete inhibition of the renin–angiotensin system would be better achieved with angiotensin II receptor antagonists or with the two drugs in combination.

INDICATIONS FOR THE USE OF ACE INHIBITORS

There are a number of compelling indications for the use of ACE inhibitors (Box 3.16).

● One indication is the presence of heart failure. Because high blood pressure is a major cause of heart failure, many patients with hypertension have co-existing heart failure. Indeed, as many as

---

Box 3.16 Indications for the use of ACE inhibitors

Heart failure
Nephropathy (diabetic and non-diabetic)
Post-myocardial infarction
High-risk patients with cardiovascular disease (HOPE)
Low-risk patients with coronary artery disease (EUROPA)

50% of the patients in some of the heart failure trials have been hypertensive.

- Nephropathy, whether diabetic or non-diabetic, is also a compelling indication for the use of ACE inhibition, because ACE inhibitors effectively reduce the rate of decline of renal function and urinary protein excretion to a greater extent than that expected by blood pressure reduction alone.
- The ACE inhibitors are also effective in normotensive patients with type 1 diabetes and microalbuminuria.

> **Important:** The ACE inhibitors are considered the drugs of choice for first-line therapy in patients with type 1 diabetes. Evidence also gives some support to the possibility that ACE inhibitors may reduce the incidence of new-onset diabetes.

CONTRA-INDICATIONS TO THE USE OF ACE INHIBITORS

> **Bilateral renal artery stenosis is a major contra-indication to the use of ACE inhibition because it may precipitate renal failure. In unilateral renal artery stenosis, ACE inhibitors should be used only under expert guidance, as again there is a risk of deterioration in renal function.**

The mechanism behind the ability of ACE inhibitors to further impair renal function in renal artery stenosis is as follows. Stenosis of the afferent renal artery leads to a decrease in glomerular filtration pressure and increased production of angiotensin II, which then maintains glomerular filtration via constriction of the efferent renal arteriole. The inhibition of angiotensin II production by ACE inhibition can thus cause a decrease in renal glomerular perfusion pressure to a level at which filtration ceases. The discontinuation of ACE inhibitor therapy and careful volume replacement usually reverses the situation, although some patients can require haemodialysis.

> **Important:** It is important to monitor urea and electrolytes in all patients around 10 days after initiation of treatment with an ACE inhibitor. A limited rise in serum creatinine of up to 35% above baseline with ACE inhibitors (or angiotensin receptor antagonists) is acceptable unless hyperkalaemia develops.[17] However, if any significant rise occurs it is wise to monitor electrolytes at regular intervals.

In fact, ACE inhibitors (or angiotensin receptor antagonists) are often effective in achieving good blood pressure control in some cases of renal artery stenosis where other drugs may have failed, particularly if the affected kidney is already contributing little to renal function but is producing high levels of renin. However, it must be emphasized that they should be used in these circumstances only under specialist supervision.

- Patients with peripheral vascular disease and diabetes should be monitored particularly closely due to the association between these conditions and renal artery stenosis.
- Patients on chronic therapy with NSAIDs are also at increased risk of renal failure, because in addition to angiotensin II, renal function is regulated by prostaglandins (the production of which is inhibited by NSAIDs). This is more likely to occur in patients with underlying renal disease. In addition, NSAIDs are known to blunt the anti-hypertensive effect of ACE inhibition.

> ⚠ ACE inhibition is *absolutely* contra-indicated in the second and third trimesters of pregnancy, and women of childbearing age should not be established on ACE inhibition without adequate contraception.

When used in the second to third trimesters of pregnancy, ACE inhibitors are associated with pulmonary hypoplasia, fetal skull hypoplasia, growth retardation, and renal failure in the fetus.[18] If a woman taking an ACE inhibitor inadvertently becomes pregnant despite the above precautions, the ACE inhibitor should be stopped as soon as possible.

ADVERSE EFFECTS OF ACE INHIBITION

In addition to the precipitation of acute renal failure in patients with renal artery stenosis or on NSAIDs, ACE inhibition has a number of other adverse effects.

The major adverse effect of ACE inhibition is ACE inhibitor-induced cough, which affects approximately 10% of individuals. Typically the cough is dry, non-productive, and not dose-related. Suggestions as to the aetiology of the cough include potentiation of bradykinin levels, increased sensitivity of the normal cough reflex, and increased circulating levels of prostaglandins. However, the cough is definitely a feature of ACE inhibition rather than the blockade of the renin–angiotensin system because angiotensin II receptor blockers do not exhibit this side effect.

> ⚠ **Angio-oedema is a rare but potentially life-threatening adverse effect of ACE inhibition. It usually occurs within several days to a week after initiation of treatment, and it is characterized by facial and lingual swelling, which can be enough to cause breathing difficulties.**

Interestingly, angio-oedema appears to be more common after treatment with combined ACE–neutral endopeptidase inhibition, especially in black Afro-Caribbean people, although the mechanism for this remains unclear.

Other adverse effects include a macular rash, which can occur in 3–5% of patients, and loss of taste and appetite. The latter is uncommon but can cause weight loss in the elderly if the condition is not recognized.

Effects on cardiovascular outcome

Blood pressure responses to ACE inhibitors are similar to those of other classes of agent, with response rates from 40 to 70%. However, certain sub-groups demonstrate lower response rates in mono-therapy with ACE inhibitors, including low-renin, salt-sensitive individuals such as diabetic and black patients.

There are no large randomized trials comparing ACE inhibition with placebo in patients with hypertension. The Captopril Prevention Project (CAPP) study compared a regimen based on the ACE inhibitor captopril with standard therapy based on diuretics and β blockade, although the design of the study has been subject to criticism. The cardiovascular outcomes were broadly equivalent between the two groups, but there were significantly more strokes in the ACE inhibitor group.[15] Another study, the Swedish Trial in Old Patients with Hypertension–2 (STOP–2), also showed no clear benefit of ACE inhibitor therapy over conventional treatment in terms of cardiovascular outcome.

In the CAPP study, individuals with type 2 diabetes had a greater reduction in cardiovascular end points than that in those receiving conventional therapy. However, this finding is not supported by results from the UK Prospective Diabetes Study in subjects with newly diagnosed type 2 diabetes. In this study, the β blocker atenolol was equally as effective as the ACE inhibitor captopril in reducing the incidence of stroke, while neither agent significantly reduced the incidence of myocardial infarction.

The Second Australian National Blood Pressure Study compared cardiovascular outcome in elderly patients following treatment with ACE inhibitors or diuretics; 6083 subjects with hypertension between the ages of 65 and 84 were studied. The authors concluded that initiation of anti-hypertensive treatment involving ACE inhibitors in older individuals, particularly men, appears to lead to a better outcome than that of treatment with diuretic agents, despite similar reductions of blood pressure. However, the design and results of this study have been subject to some criticism.

In contrast, the largest hypertension trial to date, ALLHAT, did not show any difference in outcome between the ACE inhibitor lisinopril and the diuretic chlorthalidone. In ALLHAT, there was a 15% higher stroke rate in the group treated with the ACE inhibitor, lisinopril, compared with the total study population, and in the black cohort treated with lisinopril the stroke rate was 40% higher that in the total study population. Such differences would favour a diuretic over an ACE inhibitor for stroke reduction. However, there were small differences in blood pressure between the treatment groups with systolic blood pressure being 2 mmHg higher in the lisinopril-treated patients and 4 mmHg higher in black participants.

The Perindopril Protection Against Recurrent Stroke Study (PROGRESS) reported that a combination of the ACE inhibitor perindopril and indapamide reduces recurrent stroke in both normotensive and hypertensive patients who have suffered a previous stroke. However, perindopril alone failed to reduce stroke incidence despite a 2–4 mmHg reduction in blood pressure.

Two studies, Heart Outcomes Prevention Evaluation (HOPE) and the European Trial on Reduction of Cardiac Events with Perindopril in Stable Coronary Artery Disease (EUROPA), have examined the effect of ACE inhibition in individuals with high cardiovascular risk and in lower risk individuals with coronary artery disease, respectively.

The HOPE[19] study compared the ACE inhibitor ramipril (10 mg/day) against placebo in 9297 patients at high risk of cardiovascular events. The primary composite end point was cardiovascular death, non-fatal myocardial infarction and non-fatal stroke. The trial was terminated early after 4.5 years due to a 22% relative risk reduction in the ramipril-treated group. Reductions in the individual end points were 32% for stroke, 26% for all cardiovascular death, and 20% for myocardial infarction.

The EUROPA[20] study involved 12 218 patients with stable coronary artery disease but no evidence of heart failure treated with 8 mg of the ACE inhibitor perindopril one daily or placebo. The results showed that patients receiving perindopril had a reduction of 20% in the primary end point (cardiovascular death, myocardial infarction or cardiac arrest) compared with those in the placebo group.

In contrast, the Prevention of Events with Angiotension Converting Enzyme Inhibition (PEACE) Trial[21], in patients with stable coronary artery disease and preserved left ventricular function, failed to show a difference in the incidence of the primary end point of death from cardiovascular causes, myocardial infarction or coronary revascularization, with the addition of trandolapril compared to placebo.

In summary, ACE inhibitors are probably as effective as traditional agents such as thiazide diuretics in reducing mortality in hypertensive subjects, but any superiority over other agents remains to be established.

ANGIOTENSIN RECEPTOR ANTAGONISTS

The first angiotensin receptor antagonist to be developed and released into clinical practice was losartan in 1995. Since then, several other angiotensin receptor antagonists have been developed, including:

- candesartan
- eprosartan
- irbesartan
- telmisartan
- valsartan.

Angiotensin receptor antagonists act by blocking the effects of angiotensin II on the angiotensin receptor. There are two subtypes of angiotensin receptor: AT_1 and AT_2. Angiotensin receptor antagonists act preferentially on the AT_1 subtype of receptor.

Angiotensin II is a potent vasoconstrictor and also has trophic and growth-promoting effects on tissues. Blockade of angiotensin II effects by angiotensin receptor antagonists leads to a reduction in blood pressure and may also have beneficial effects on the myocardium in heart failure and on the kidneys in diabetic nephropathy or microalbuminuria.

Unlike the action of ACE inhibitors, blockade of the pathway at the level of the angiotensin receptor does not cause accumulation of bradykinin, thought to be the mechanism of the ACE inhibitor-induced cough, although it may contribute to the blood pressure-lowering effects of ACE inhibitors. Also, angiotensin receptor antagonists may provide a more complete blockade of the renin–angiotensin–aldosterone system than that of ACE inhibitors because—in addition to the classical pathway of generation of angiotensin II from angiotensin I by ACE—an alternative pathway exists using chymase as an enzyme; therefore ACE inhibitors cannot fully prevent the formation of angiotensin II.

The more complete blockade produced by angiotensin receptor antagonists does not seem to confer a clinical advantage. In fact, increasingly, angiotensin receptor antagonists are being used in combination with ACE inhibitors to achieve a greater degree of block of the renin–angiotensin–aldosterone system.

TOLERABILITY

Angiotensin receptor antagonists are effective in lowering blood pressure when administered once daily due to their long duration of action. They are generally well tolerated, with few side effects.

> ⚠️ **Angiotensin receptor antagonists are contra-indicated in pregnancy due to probable fetotoxicity, and they should be used only with extreme caution in renal artery stenosis.**

As mono-therapy, angiotensin receptor antagonists tend to be more effective in younger patients, who tend to have a higher renin form of hypertension. They tend to be used as an alternative to ACE inhibitors in patients with ACE inhibitor-induced cough.

EFFICACY

Angiotensin receptor antagonists have been shown in clinical trials to be at least as effective as β blockers, calcium channel blockers, thiazide diuretics and ACE inhibitors in lowering blood pressure.

The LIFE study compared losartan with atenolol in 9193 hypertensive patients with left ventricular hypertrophy.[11] The primary end point was cardiovascular morbidity and mortality (a composite end point of cardiovascular death, myocardial infarction and stroke). The relative risk of cardiovascular morbidity and mortality was 0.87 (95% CI 0.77–0.98) in the losartan group compared with the atenolol group (Fig. 3.9), despite similar decreases in peripheral blood pressure in the two groups.

The LIFE study was the first large trial to show a significant difference in outcome between two anti-hypertensive agents. The difference in outcome may be partially explained by small baseline differences in blood pressure, and particularly pulse pressure, between the two groups, as well as the possible different effects on aortic blood pressure of the two agents, which are not necessarily reflected in measurements of blood pressure taken conventionally in the upper arm. However, the authors conclude that losartan seems to confer benefits beyond reduction in blood pressure in this study. Further outcome data for the other angiotensin receptor antagonists are awaited.

α BLOCKERS

α Blockers were first developed in the 1960s. They act by inhibiting the post-synaptic α_1 adrenoceptors on the vascular walls, which mediate increases in arterial and venous tone secondary to noradrenaline release from sympathetic nerve endings. α Blockers therefore cause peripheral vasodilatation and lower the blood pressure. Available agents include the α_1-selective agents prazosin, doxazosin, indoramin and terazosin, and the non-selective agents phenoxybenzamine and phentolamine, which are rarely used except in the pre- and peri-operative management of phaeochromocytoma.

> **Important:** α Blockers are rarely a first-choice treatment in hypertension, except in the situation of a man with hypertension and prostatism. In addition to lowering the blood pressure, they improve urinary flow rates in benign prostatic hypertrophy.

α Blockers also have small beneficial effects on cholesterol, triglyceride and HDL levels, although these are unlikely to be significant clinically.

Important: α Blockers are often used as part of combination therapy in patients who are already taking at least one other anti-hypertensive agent or in patients who have been intolerant of a number of other agents.

ADVERSE EFFECTS

Side effects of α blockers include:

- postural hypotension
- tachycardia
- dizziness
- ankle oedema
- worsening of stress incontinence
- gastrointestinal upset.

Important: α Blockers should be avoided in patients with urinary incontinence.

USE OF α BLOCKERS IN HYPERTENSION

Although α blockers are successful in lowering blood pressure, there are no good outcome data for their use in hypertension. A doxazosin treatment arm was included in ALLHAT;[2] however, the doxazosin arm was stopped early due to an apparent excess of heart failure compared with the other treatment arms using lisinopril, chlorthalidone and amlodipine.

CENTRALLY ACTING AGENTS

Centrally acting anti-hypertensive agents act on the vasomotor centres in the brain. Their main action is as α_2 agonists in the brain stem, stimulating inhibitory neurones and reducing sympathetic outflow; this leads to a reduction in peripheral vascular resistance and cardiac output, reducing blood pressure. Available agents include α-

methyldopa, clonidine and moxonidine. The latter two also have imidazoline (I_1) receptor agonist effects that lead to a further reduction in sympathetic outflow.

Centrally acting agents are not commonly used but have a place in the management of resistant hypertension in:

- patients who have experienced side effects to several of the major classes of anti-hypertensive drugs
- patients with type 1 diabetes.

α-Methyldopa is still commonly used in the treatment of hypertension and pre-eclampsia during pregnancy. It is a pro-drug and is metabolized to its active metabolite α-methylnoradrenaline.

 Clonidine is associated with severe hypertension on withdrawal of therapy and should therefore be withdrawn gradually.

Moxonidine has a more favourable side effect profile than the other agents due to a relatively lower affinity for α_2 adrenoceptors. It may also have some glucose-lowering effects in patients with the metabolic syndrome of hypertension, hyperlipidaemia and glucose intolerance.

There are no good outcome data for the use of these drugs in hypertension.

ADVERSE EFFECTS

 Side-effects of centrally acting agents are common and include drowsiness and depression. They should be avoided in patients who drive or who operate machinery.

Centrally acting agents cause:

- dry mouth
- dizziness
- fatigue
- headaches
- vivid dreams.

Generally these agents are much less well tolerated than the more commonly used classes of anti-hypertensive agents, and compliance is a major problem.

ARTERIAL VASODILATORS

Arterial vasodilators are rarely used as first-line agents and tend to be reserved for resistant cases of hypertension that have failed to respond to other more commonly used drugs. They are particularly effective in patients with hypertension mainly due to increased peripheral vascular resistance.

The three drugs that are available are hydralazine, minoxidil and diazoxide.

- The mechanism of action of hydralazine is not known, but it appears to act as a direct arterial vasodilator. Hydralazine is rarely used, although it still has an occasional role in the management of hypertension in pregnancy because it is thought to be safe for the fetus.
- Minoxidil is a potent arterial vasodilator and acts as a potassium channel opener. It is used occasionally in patients with resistant hypertension whose condition has failed to respond to other drugs. It is usually given in combination with a loop diuretic to reduce fluid retention and a β blocker to control the reflex tachycardia that it induces.
- Diazoxide is also a potassium channel opener and a very potent vasodilator. It was previously used to control hypertension in patients having renal dialysis but is rarely used now.

There are no outcome data for the use of the arterial vasodilators in hypertension.

ADVERSE EFFECTS

The side effects of the arterial vasodilators are mainly due to physiological counter-regulatory mechanisms stimulated by the profound vasodilatation induced by these agents. Baroreceptors are activated, leading to increased sympathetic outflow, reflex tachycardia, and increased plasma catecholamine levels. Salt and water retention occurs, which limits the usefulness of these agents in lowering blood pressure. Patients also commonly experience headache and flushing due to the vasodilator effects of the drugs.

> ⚠ **Arterial vasodilators should be avoided as mono-therapy in patients with angina because these drugs may worsen the condition due to an increase in heart rate.**

Hydralazine has been associated with a dose-dependent, lupus-like syndrome presenting as fever, rash and arthralgia, which usually resolves on stopping the drug. Positive antinuclear antibodies occur in up to 40% of patients on treatment with hydralazine. The metabolism of hydralazine shows a genetic bimodal distribution with fast and slow acetylator genotypes. Patients with the slow acetylator genotype are more likely to develop the lupus-like syndrome with hydralazine.

Minoxidil causes excess hair growth, mainly on the limbs and face, which is particularly troublesome for female patients, who may find it necessary to shave facial hair. Due to this effect, it is also marketed as a topical treatment for male pattern baldness.

Diazoxide is structurally similar to the thiazide diuretics, and like the thiazides may elevate glucose levels.

OTHER AGENTS

Certain drugs that are available for other indications may also have a role in the treatment of hypertension.

NITRATES

Long-acting nitrates such as isosorbide mononitrate (modified release) act on both the arteries and the veins, causing dilatation. They have relatively greater effect on the large arteries, and this may result in a reduction of large artery stiffness, which is thought to be the primary underlying abnormality responsible for isolated systolic hypertension. Nitrates may therefore have a place in the management of this type of hypertension.

NICORANDIL

Nicorandil is used as an anti-anginal agent; however, it also has a small but significant effect on lowering blood pressure. In addition to its potassium channel-opening effects, it also contains a nitro group that activates guanidyl cyclase directly, causing vasodilatation.

THIAZOLIDINEDIONES

The thiazolidinediones (peroxisome-proliferating activating receptor-γ agonists) rosiglitazone and pioglitazone, which are used in the treatment of type 2 diabetes mellitus, have some action in lowering blood pressure. Although they are not licensed for this indication, it is a useful effect in patients who are taking them for diabetes, because many of these patients will have co-existing hypertension.

RENIN INHIBITORS

In addition to new agents that are being developed in the currently established drug classes, other agents with novel mechanisms of action may also become useful in treating hypertension. Renin inhibitors are being developed at present. Some of the most promising ones so far are analogues of angiotensinogen; however, low oral bioavailability has been a problem.

ENDOTHELIN ANTAGONISTS

Endothelin antagonists may also be useful in lowering blood pressure. Endothelin-1 is a potent vasoconstrictor acting at ET_A receptors. Bosentan is an oral competitive antagonist at ET_A and ET_B receptors, leading to a reduction in peripheral vascular resistance. It is licensed for use in pulmonary hypertension but its effects in systemic hypertension have been disappointing. Its use is also limited by its potential to cause disturbances in liver function, and it is very expensive.

NEUTRAL ENDOPEPTIDASE INHIBITORS

Neutral endopeptidase is the major enzyme involved in degrading natriuretic peptides. Neutral endopeptidase inhibitors cause elevation of the levels of atrial natriuretic peptide, bradykinin and other peptides. Although relatively ineffective in lowering blood pressure used alone, they may have greater potential for effectiveness when combined with other agents, such as ACE inhibitors or endothelin-converting enzyme inhibitors.

Omipatrilat is a combined neutral endopeptidase inhibitor and ACE inhibitor (also known as a vasopeptidase or dual inhibitor) that has shown some promising results in patients with hypertension. However, like ACE inhibitors it can cause cough and angio-oedema. Other similar agents are under development.

REFERENCES

1. Pickkers P, Hughes AD, Russel FG, et al. Thiazide-induced vasodilation in humans is mediated by potassium channel activation. Hypertension 1998; 32(6): 1071–1076.

2. Major outcomes in high-risk hypertensive patients randomized to angiotensin-converting enzyme inhibitor or calcium channel blocker vs diuretic: the Antihypertensive and Lipid-Lowering Treatment to Prevent Heart Attack Trial (ALLHAT). JAMA 2002; 288(23): 2981–2997.

3. SHEP Cooperative Research Group. Prevention of stroke by antihypertensive drug treatment in older persons with isolated systolic hypertension: final results of the Systolic Hypertension in the Elderly Program. JAMA 1991; 265: 3255–3265.

4. Cockcroft JR. Nebivolol: more than just another beta-blocker? Prescriber 1999; 5.

5. Medical Research Council Working Party. MRC trial of treatment of mild hypertension: principal results. Br Med J (Clin Res Ed) 1985; 291(6488): 97–104.

6. Materson BJ, Reda DJ, Cushman WC, et al. Single-drug therapy for hypertension in men. A comparison of six antihypertensive agents with placebo. The Department of Veterans Affairs Cooperative Study Group on Antihypertensive Agents. N Engl J Med 1993; 328(13): 914–921.

7. Philipp T, Anlauf M, Distler A, et al. Randomised, double blind, multicentre comparison of hydrochlorothiazide, atenolol, nitrendipine, and enalapril in antihypertensive treatment: results of the HANE study. HANE Trial Research Group. Br Med J 1997; 315(7101): 154–159.

8. Messerli FH, Beevers DG, Franklin SS, et al. Beta-blockers in hypertension—the emperor has no clothes: an open letter to present and prospective drafters of new guidelines for the treatment of hypertension. Am J Hypertens 2003; 16(10): 870–873.

9. MRC Working Party. Medical Research Council trial of treatment of hypertension in older adults: principal results. Br Med J 1992; 304(6824): 405–412.

10. Messerli FH, Grossman E, Goldbourt U. Are beta-blockers efficacious as first-line therapy for hypertension in the elderly? A systematic review. JAMA 1998; 279(23): 1903–1907.

11. Dahlof B, Devereux RB, Kjeldsen SE, et al. Cardiovascular morbidity and mortality in the Losartan Intervention For Endpoint reduction in hypertension study (LIFE): a randomised trial against atenolol. Lancet 2002; 359(9311): 995–1003.

12. SB. Propranolol and depression: evidence from the antihypertensive trials. Can J Psychiatry 1990; 35(3): 257–259.

13. Packer M, O'Connor CM, Ghali JK, et al. Effect of amlodipine on morbidity and mortality in severe chronic heart failure. Prospective Randomized Amlodipine Survival Evaluation Study Group. N Engl J Med 1996; 335(15): 1107–1114.

14. Brown MJ, Palmer CR, Castaigne A, et al. Morbidity and mortality in patients randomised to double-blind treatment with a long-acting calcium-

channel blocker or diuretic in the International Nifedipine GITS study: Intervention as a Goal in Hypertension Treatment (INSIGHT). Lancet 2000; 356(9227): 366–372.

15. Hansson L, Lindholm LH, Ekbom T, et al. Randomised trial of old and new antihypertensive drugs in elderly patients: cardiovascular mortality and morbidity in the Swedish Trial in Old Patients with Hypertension–2 study. Lancet 1999; 354(9192): 1751–1756.

16. Staessen JA, Wang JG, Thijs L. Cardiovascular protection and blood pressure reduction: a meta-analysis. Lancet 2001; 358(9290): 1305–1315.

17. Chobanian AV, Bakris GL, Black HR, et al. The Seventh Report of the Joint National Committee on Prevention, Detection, Evaluation, and Treatment of High Blood Pressure: the JNC 7 report. JAMA 2003; 289(19): 2560–2572.

18. Briggs GG. Medication use during the perinatal period. J Am Pharm Assoc (Wash) 1998; 38(6): 717–726.

19. Yusuf S, Sleight P, Pogue J, et al. Effects of an angiotensin-converting enzyme inhibitor, ramipril, on cardiovascular events in high-risk patients. The Heart Outcomes Prevention Evaluation Study Investigators. N Engl J Med 2003; 342(3): 145–153.

20. Fox KM. European trial On Reduction of cardiac events with Perindopril in stable coronary Artery disease Investigators. Efficacy of cardiovascular events among patients with stable coronary artery disease; randomised, double-blind, placebo-controlled, multicentre trial. Lancet 2003; 362(9386): 782–788.

21. Braunwald E, Domanski MJ, Fowler SE, et al. Angiotensisn-converting enzyme inhibition in stable coronary artery disease. N Engl J Med 2004; 351(20): 2058–2068.

OTHER
INTERVENTIONS

In addition to blood pressure-lowering medication, other pharmaco-logical interventions may improve outcome in hypertensive patients. The current British Hypertension Society guidelines for the use of statins and aspirin in hypertension are summarized in Box 3.17, and the evidence for their use is discussed further below. There is no good evidence supporting the use of vitamins in hypertension.

LIPID-LOWERING THERAPY

Several studies have demonstrated the benefits of lipid-lowering therapy for the primary and secondary prevention of cardiovascular disease. Significant reductions in myocardial infarction, stroke and mortality of up to around 30% have been described.

Box 3.17 Guidelines for the use of aspirin and statins in hypertensive patients

Primary prevention
Aspirin
Use 75 mg daily if the patient is aged ≥50 years with blood pressure controlled to <150/90 mmHg and target organ damage, diabetes mellitus, or 10-year risk of cardiovascular disease of ≥20% (measured using the Joint British Societies' cardiovascular disease risk chart, available through http://www.bhsoc.org).

Statin
Use sufficient doses to reach targets if the patient is aged up to at least 80 years with a 10-year cardiovascular risk of ≥20% and total cholesterol concentration ≥3.5 mmol/L.

Secondary prevention (including for patients with type 2 diabetes)
Aspirin
Use for all patients unless contra-indicated.

Statin
Use sufficient doses to reach targets if the patient is aged up to at least 80 years with a total cholesterol concentration ≥3.5 mmol/L.

(After Williams et al 2004,[1] Br Med J; 328:634–640 with permission from the BMJ Publishing Group.)

Two of the early keystone trials were the West of Scotland Coronary Prevention Study (WOSCOPS),[2] a primary prevention trial using pravastatin, and the Scandinavian Simvastatin Survival Study (4S),[3] a secondary prevention trial using simvastatin. More recently, the MRC–British Heart Foundation Heart Protection Study (HPS) showed that in 20 536 high-risk patients, treatment with simvastatin 40 mg daily significantly reduced vascular events and all-cause mortality, largely irrespective of initial cholesterol concentrations.[4]

Hypertension and hypercholesterolaemia often co-exist as risk factors, and two recent studies have looked at the benefits of lipid-lowering therapy in hypertensive patients.

Because hypertensive patients are at higher absolute risk of vascular events, one might expect that they would benefit from lipid-lowering therapy at least to the same degree or more than non-hypertensive patients. However, the Antihypertensive and Lipid-Lowering Treatment to Prevent Heart Attack Trial (ALLHAT–LLT) failed to demonstrate a significant difference in all-cause mortality between those patients treated with pravastatin or usual care in a group of 10 355 moderately hypercholesterolaemic, hypertensive patients.[5] This may have been due to the large number of patients in the 'usual care' arm who received statins and the choice of agent used, resulting in a small differential in total cholesterol between the two study arms.

In contrast to ALLHAT–LLT, the Anglo-Scandinavian Cardiac Outcomes Trial–Lipid Lowering Arm (ASCOT–LLA) showed that in 10 305 hypertensive patients with average or lower than average cholesterol levels, treatment with atorvastatin significantly reduced major cardiovascular events.

A number of epidemiological studies have suggested that there is a relationship between blood pressure and cholesterol levels, and that the reduction of cholesterol can lead to a reduction in blood pressure.[6] A meta-analysis of lipid-lowering trials showed that treatment with statins reduces the incidence of stroke by around 32%. Because there is clear evidence of a link between blood pressure and stroke, and blood pressure reduction results in a similar (40%) reduction in stroke, these findings suggest that cholesterol reduction may prevent stroke via a decrease in blood pressure. Indeed, the hypotensive effect of statin therapy was demonstrated in a study using pravastatin in patients with hypertension and hypercholesterolaemia.[7]

Although the greatest body of outcome evidence exists for the statins, other lipid-lowering therapies may also be useful in hypertensive patients, particularly in those who are intolerant of statins or whose condition fails to respond adequately to reasonable doses of statins. Such alternatives include:

- the fibrates
- ezetimibe.

Ezetimibe reduces cholesterol absorption from the gastrointestinal tract.

ASPIRIN

There is some contention over the value of aspirin treatment in hypertensive patients. The Thrombosis Prevention Trial was a placebo-controlled study of the effects of 75 mg aspirin daily or warfarin; 26% of the study population were hypertensive.[8] Aspirin led to a 16% reduction in all cardiovascular events and a 20% reduction in myocardial infarction, but it had no effect on fatal events. The number of events prevented was offset by similar rates of bleeding events. These findings were similar to those of an arm of the Hypertension Optimal Treatment (HOT) study, which compared 75 mg aspirin daily with placebo.[9] Most bleeding events occurred in patients with particularly high systolic blood pressure.

Current recommendations are that blood pressure should be controlled to at least less than 150/90 mmHg before aspirin is used.

REFERENCES

1. Williams B, Poulter NR, Brown MJ, et al. British Hypertension Society guidelines for hypertension management 2004 (BHS-IV): summary. Br Med J 2004; 328: 634–640.
2. Influence of pravastatin and plasma lipids on clinical events in the West of Scotland Coronary Prevention Study (WOSCOPS). Circulation 1998; 97: 1440–1445.
3. Scandinavian Simvastatin Survival Study Group. Randomized trial of cholesterol lowering in 4444 patients with coronary heart disease: the Scandinavian Simvastatin Survival Study (4S). Lancet 1995; 344: 1383–1389.
4. Heart Protection Study Collaborative Group. MRC/BHF Heart Protection Study of cholesterol lowering with simvastatin in 20,536 high-risk individuals: a randomised placebo-controlled trial. Lancet 2002; 360(9326): 7–22.

5. Major outcomes in moderately hypercholesterolemic, hypertensive patients randomized to pravastatin vs usual care: the Antihypertensive and Lipid-Lowering Treatment to Prevent Heart Attack Trial (ALLHAT–LLT). JAMA 2002; 288(23): 2998–3007.

6. Goode GK, Miller JP, Heagerty AM. Hyperlipidaemia, hypertension, and coronary heart disease. Lancet 1995; 354: 362–364.

7. Glorioso N, Troffa C, Filigheddu F, et al. Effect of the HMG-CoA reductase inhibitors on blood pressure in patients with essential hypertension and primary hypercholesterolemia. Hypertension 2000; 34: 1281–1286.

8. Thrombosis Prevention Trial: randomised trial of low-intensity oral anticoagulation with warfarin and low-dose aspirin in the primary prevention of ischaemic heart disease in men at increased risk. The Medical Research Council's General Practice Research Framework. Lancet 1998; 351(9098): 233–241.

9. Hansson L, Zanchetti A, Carruthers SG, et al. Effects of intensive blood-pressure lowering and low-dose aspirin in patients with hypertension: principal results of the Hypertension Optimal Treatment (HOT) randomised trial. HOT Study Group. Lancet 1998; 351(9118): 1755–1762.

CHAPTER 4

TREATMENT OF HYPERTENSION IN SPECIAL PATIENT GROUPS

MALIGNANT HYPERTENSION

Although once relatively common, malignant hypertension is today rare in Westernized countries. It remains, however, a potentially life-threatening condition that is frequently poorly managed. Untreated, it carries a 90% 5-year mortality. With adequate treatment this figure has been reduced to less than 20%.

The hallmark of malignant hypertension is severe hypertension with bilateral retinal haemorrhages, with or without papilloedema (Fig. 4.1). The diastolic pressure is usually, but not always, greater than 120 mmHg. Unlike those with essential hypertension, patients with malignant hypertension frequently have symptoms and signs related to the marked blood pressure elevation including, for example, headache and blurred vision; see Box 1.1 (p. 14) and Table 1.3 (p. 14) for a comprehensive list. Likewise, end-organ damage is often severe at presentation, and patients may present with cardiac or renal failure (see Box 1.2, p. 15).

Hypertensive emergencies are listed in Box 4.1. Patients require:

- immediate admission, often to the intensive care unit
- intravenous therapy to reduce the blood pressure to a safe level.

Box 4.1 Hypertensive emergencies

Hypertensive encephalopathy
Hypertensive heart failure
Hypertension with aortic dissection
Severe pre-eclampsia or eclampsia
Phaeochromocytoma crisis

The following acts as a guide, but local practices differ. The key is a controlled reduction in blood pressure.

Important: The most important point regarding the management of malignant hypertension is to distinguish between those patients with a hypertensive emergency and those who need urgent treatment (a situation often, unfortunately, called 'hypertensive urgency').

 There is absolutely no substitute for the direct involvement of a senior clinician experienced in the management of malignant hypertension.

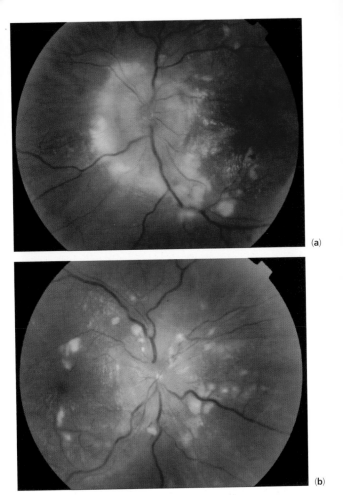

(a)

(b)

Fig. 4.1 Retinal appearances in malignant hypertension. There is gross papilloedema with flame-shaped retinal haemorrhages, hard exudates and soft exudates characteristic of retinal ischaemia in both the right (**a**) and left (**b**) eyes in this patient with malignant hypertension.

HYPERTENSIVE ENCEPHALOPATHY

Hypertensive encephalopathy refers to malignant hypertension with signs of cerebral oedema including coma or seizures. This may be confirmed using computerized tomography or magnetic resonance imaging.

The classical drug of choice is intravenous sodium nitroprusside.

- Sodium nitroprusside is a very potent, directly acting vasodilator that must be shielded from light.
- Its use requires insertion of an intra-arterial line for accurate blood pressure monitoring because its effects are rapid, profound and short-lived.
- The dose must be adjusted carefully and titrated against the fall in blood pressure.
- Sodium nitroprusside has a toxic metabolite that may lead to cyanide or thiocyanate toxicity with prolonged use; this may be prevented by the concomitant administration of hydroxocobalamin.

Intravenous glyceryl trinitrate or labetalol are alternatives that have been used successfully.

> ⚠ **Very abrupt reductions in blood pressure should be avoided, and the immediate goal should be to reduce the diastolic pressure to around 110 mmHg. Thereafter a much more gradual reduction in pressure should be the aim.**

HYPERTENSIVE HEART FAILURE

Treatment for hypertensive heart failure should be as for classical left ventricular failure, with the addition of intravenous sodium nitroprusside or glyceryl trinitrate.

HYPERTENSION WITH AORTIC DISSECTION

The aim is to reduce the blood pressure to a systolic pressure of 110 mmHg and slow the heart rate. Intravenous labetalol is usually the drug of choice, given with or without a nitrate such as glyceryl trinitrate.

SEVERE PRE-ECLAMPSIA OR ECLAMPSIA

The ultimate aim is the safe delivery of the fetus, usually as an emergency Caesarean section. Magnesium sulphate should be given intravenously.

 The aim in terms of blood pressure should be a controlled reduction in diastolic pressure to around 100 mmHg. Abrupt reductions must be avoided.

Intravenous hydralazine or labetalol may be used with volume replacement as necessary. Nitroprusside may be required in refractory cases.

PHAEOCHROMOCYTOMA CRISIS

The drug of choice is the intravenous α-adrenoceptor antagonist phentolamine.

OTHER PATIENTS

For the remainder of patients with malignant hypertension, oral therapy is indicated. Most but not all patients require admission to hospital to monitor the response to therapy and initiate further investigations.

The standard first-line therapy is a β blocker, such as atenolol 25–50 mg daily. A reasonable alternative is **modified-release** nifedipine 10–20 mg daily.

 The aim is to reduce the blood pressure by 20–30 mmHg daily; more rapid reductions in blood pressure are associated with cerebral hypoperfusion and stroke. Short-acting agents such as standard nifedipine MUST NOT be used under any circumstances.

In patients with fluid overload, loop diuretics may be indicated. Later on in therapy, a reasonable combination is a β blocker and a calcium channel blocker.

DIABETES AND HYPERTENSION

PREVALENCE OF HYPERTENSION IN DIABETES

Hypertension is twice as common in individuals with diabetes as in those who are non-diabetic. In white populations, hypertension affects 10–30% of patients with type 1 diabetes and 20–40% of those with impaired glucose tolerance.

The exact prevalence of hypertension in individuals with type 2 diabetes will vary depending on the values of systolic and diastolic blood pressure used to define hypertension.

- Using the definition of systolic blood pressure at least 160 mmHg and diastolic blood pressure at least 95 mmHg, the prevalence of hypertension in individuals over 55 years of age with type 2 diabetes is 43% in men and 52% in women (Hypertension in Diabetes study, 1993).
- In the UK Prospective Diabetes Study (UKPDS), the prevalence of hypertension in newly diagnosed type 2 diabetic patients was 39%.
- If a systolic pressure of at least 140 and/or diastolic pressure of at least 90 mmHg is used, approximately 80% of type 2 diabetic patients are hypertensive in some series.

Hypertension associated with diabetes probably accounts for up to 85% of excess risk of cardiovascular disease. In addition, patients with hypertension are more prone to diabetes than are normotensive individuals. The increased cardiovascular risk associated with type 2 diabetes may also be due to clustering of other risk factors with diabetes in the metabolic syndrome (Box 4.2).

Box 4.2 Components of the metabolic syndrome commonly associated with type 2 diabetes mellitus

Microalbuminuria
Obesity
Insulin resistance
Dyslipidaemia (increased triglycerides and small dense LDL cholesterol particles)
Hypercoagulation
Inflammation
Left ventricular hypertrophy
Hyperuricaemia

MECHANISMS OF HYPERTENSION IN DIABETES MELLITUS

The exact mechanisms involved in the genesis of hypertension in individuals with diabetes remain to be elucidated.

As in those without diabetes, individuals with diabetes can develop essential hypertension coincidentally, and this is believed to account for around 10% of hypertension in the diabetic population. Genetic factors play a role in the genesis of hypertension in the general population; these factors may also be involved in the development of insulin resistance and thus increase the risk of developing type 2 diabetes. Indeed, it has been suggested that genetic and environmental factors operating in the fetal stage and in early infancy may be involved in the genesis of both hypertension and diabetes. Other possible mechanisms are listed in Box 4.3.

The normal age-related rise in blood pressure is exaggerated in patients with type 2 diabetes. This is due to premature vascular ageing, which may be due to factors such as endothelial dysfunction and/or vascular inflammation, leading to increased arterial stiffening. Such changes may account for the fact that isolated systolic hypertension, a condition characterized by large arterial stiffening, is more common in patients with type 2 diabetes.

Patients with type 2 diabetes are insulin-resistant, and insulin has been shown to have a beneficial effect in that it decreases large arterial stiffness, an effect that is blunted in obese insulin-resistant individuals.

A number of endocrine causes of hypertension may co-exist with diabetes, including thyrotoxicosis, Cushing's syndrome, phaeochromocytoma and acromegaly. Therefore the possibility of a secondary cause of hypertension should always be considered in patients with diabetes, especially renal artery stenosis, which is more common in the diabetic population.

Box 4.3 Possible mechanisms associated with the development of hypertension in diabetes

Increased sodium reabsorption
Increased contractility of vascular smooth muscle
Increased activity of the sympathetic nervous system
Endothelial dysfunction
Diabetic nephropathy

TREATMENT TARGETS IN DIABETES MELLITUS

The major cause of death and morbidity in individuals with diabetes is cardiovascular disease, and the object of therapy for hypertension in patients with diabetes is a significant reduction of cardiovascular morbidity and mortality. Therefore all cardiovascular risk factors must be controlled concomitantly. This is important because, in a similar way as with blood pressure itself, there appears to be no threshold of risk for the other common risk factors such as hypercholesterolaemia and hyperglycaemia. Treatment and treatment targets for blood pressure will therefore depend to some extent on whether the individual is at a high or low overall cardiovascular risk.

MICROVASCULAR COMPLICATIONS

Of those patients with long-standing type 1 diabetes, approximately 40–50% will develop significant microvascular disease (retinopathy, nephropathy or neuropathy). Although type 2 diabetic individuals have a greater risk of macrovascular disease than those with type 1 diabetes, microvascular disease is becoming increasingly recognized in the type 2 diabetic population. Unlike macrovascular complications of diabetes, which are not directly related to hyperglycaemia or duration of diabetes, the duration and severity of diabetes do influence the overall development of microvascular disease; other factors that influence the susceptibility of a particular individual remain unclear.

DIABETIC NEPHROPATHY

The risk of developing diabetic nephropathy appears to be similar in patients with type 1 and type 2 diabetes. However, the incidence of diabetic nephropathy is higher in black patients than in white patients. Again, the mechanisms involved are not as yet known. Clustering of nephropathy cases suggests a genetic basis in some patient groups.

Approximately 8% of type 2 diabetic individuals will develop early nephropathy as manifest by microalbuminuria 1–3 years after diagnosis. The prevalence of microalbuminuria rises to 50–60% after 20–30 years of diabetes.

Patients with microalbuminuria have a significantly increased risk of cardiovascular disease and also the subsequent development of frank proteinuria. Indeed, approximately 50% of patients with microalbuminuria will progress to develop proteinuria. There is a very high mortality in patients with proteinuria, and median survival is approximately 10 years in such patients.

The transition from micro- to frank proteinuria appears to be influenced by glycaemic control. In the UKPDS, whereas tight glycaemic control was not very effective in reducing macrovascular disease, both tight glycaemic control and tight blood pressure control were effective in reducing microvascular complications.

DIABETIC RETINOPATHY

The prevalence of diabetic retinopathy is greatest in early-onset type 1 diabetic patients and lowest in diabetic patients not being treated with insulin. In all cases the prevalence increases with age. Diabetic retinopathy is present in 25% of individuals after 15 years of diabetes and 50% after 20 years. In older-onset individuals, the 10-year incidence of proliferative retinopathy is 8–11%, even in those with diabetes of less than 5 years' duration.

In the UKPDS, tight blood pressure control was better than tight glycaemic control in reducing the incidence of diabetic retinopathy.

Proliferative retinopathy is caused by the formation of abnormal new blood vessels that grow from the retina into the pre-retinal space, in the vitreous, and occasionally in the iris (rubeosis iridis). New vessels appear as networks of fine branching vessels overlying the normal retinal vessels and arising from the vein (Fig. 4.2).

DIABETIC NEUROPATHY

Diabetes causes a variety of neuropathies. These tend to be related to the duration of diabetes, and they include segmental diffuse and predominantly sensory neuropathy and a small-fibre form commonly associated with autonomic neuropathy. Acute reversible neuropathies include mononeuropathies that affect individual nerves, including cranial nerves, and painful peripheral neuropathies. Distal symmetrical neuropathy probably affects 20–30% of individuals with diabetes, and the incidence and extent increase with the duration and severity of the disease.

MACROVASCULAR COMPLICATIONS

Macrovascular disease is due to atheroma and is several-fold more common in individuals with diabetes relative to those without.

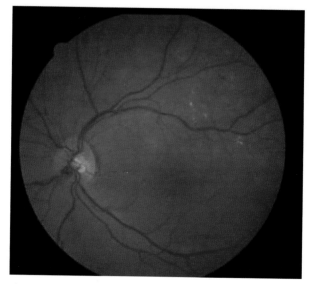

Fig. 4.2 Background diabetic retinopathy: note the presence of microaneurysms, haemorrhages and hard exudates.

Overall, the age-adjusted mortality for coronary heart disease is between two and four times higher in individuals with diabetes compared with those in control groups. Pre-menopausal women who become diabetic lose their protection against cardiovascular disease, and women with diabetes have a relatively greater excess cardiovascular risk than men. Furthermore, individuals with diabetes and angiographic evidence of coronary artery disease have a significantly worse survival rate than that of non-diabetic people. Together, this may explain to some extent the fact that individuals with diabetes have not followed the general trend of a fall in cardiovascular mortality that has been seen in the general population.

The above data mostly involve patients with type 2 diabetes. Interestingly, until recently, type 2 diabetes was regarded by some as a mild form of diabetes and essentially benign. This was especially true among the general public. However, the risk of cardiovascular disease is greater in individuals with type 2 diabetes than in those with type 1.

> **Important:** Type 2 diabetes can no longer be viewed as benign, and it should be treated as a vascular disease carrying an unacceptably high risk of heart attack and stroke.

The above view is supported by data demonstrating that mortality from coronary heart disease in patients with type 2 diabetes who have not had a myocardial infarction is the same as that in non-diabetic individuals post-myocardial infarction (Fig. 4.3).[1]

MECHANISMS OF MACROVASCULAR DISEASE

The increased risk of macrovascular disease associated with diabetes cannot be explained solely on the basis of clustering of other risk factors. There is therefore much debate as to whether diabetes itself or some other as yet unknown risk factor is responsible. Macrovascular disease correlates weakly with the level of glycaemic control or the duration of diabetes, suggesting that some other factor rather than hyperglycaemia is mediating the increased risk. The fact that many risk factors for cardiovascular disease are present long before the development of diabetes has led to the increasing support for the 'common soil' hypothesis, in which type 2 diabetes and cardiovascular disease share common genetic and environmental antecedents.[2]

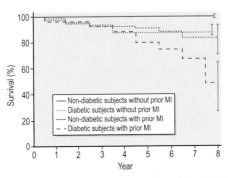

Fig. 4.3 Coronary heart disease mortality in patients with and without type 2 diabetes and myocardial infarction. (From Haffner et al © 1998,[1])

> **Box 4.4 Possible mechanisms relating hyperinsulinaemia to macrovascular disease**
>
> Increased synthesis of cholesterol
> Increased binding of LDL cholesterol
> Increased VLDL synthesis in the liver, causing increased triglycerides
> Smooth muscle hypertrophy leading to arterial wall thickening
> Increased activity of the sympathetic nervous system
> Increased release of catecholamines
> Increased sodium retention
> Inhibition of fibrinolysis due to increased hepatic production of plasminogen activator-1

Because insulin resistance leading to hyperinsulinaemia may predispose to both diabetes and cardiovascular disease, there has been much interest in the possible atherogenic actions of insulin (Box 4.4).

Microalbuminuria and proteinuria are strong and reliable markers of increased cardiovascular risk in patients with diabetes. However, non-diabetics with microalbuminuria are also at increased cardiovascular risk, suggesting that microalbuminuria is an independent risk factor for cardiovascular disease and is a marker for endothelial injury that can initiate the atheromatous process.

Data from the Steno2 trial show that multiple risk factor intervention in patients with type 2 diabetes can reduce the risk of cardiovascular events by 50%.[3]

TREATMENT OF CARDIOVASCULAR DISEASE IN PEOPLE WITH DIABETES

Acute myocardial infarction is associated with both increased acute and delayed mortality in individuals with diabetes relative to non-diabetic control subjects. A possible reason suggested for this was a reduced effect of thrombolysis in those with diabetes. However, sub-group analyses of large trials of thrombolytic therapy, which included diabetic patients, have found no evidence to support this suggestion. Indeed, thrombolysis is highly effective in patients with diabetes, and risks of intra-ocular bleeding in individuals with proliferative retinopathy are low.

Hyperglycaemia has been related to poor prognosis post myocardial infarction in individuals with diabetes, and the DIGAMI study showed that glucose and insulin therapy after acute myocardial

infarction in diabetes is associated with a significant reduction in
1-year mortality relative to control subjects.[4]

CHOICE OF DRUG THERAPY

A number of studies have shown benefit from blood pressure
reduction in diabetic patients, including the UKPDS[5] and the
Hypertension Optimal Treatment (HOT) study.[6] Indeed, in the
UKPDS, which used the β blocker atenolol and the angiotensin-
converting enzyme (ACE) inhibitor captopril, tight blood pressure
control was more effective than tight glycaemic control in reducing
macrovascular events.

Some small studies conducted in diabetic patients, such as the
Fosinopril Versus Amlodipine Cardiovascular Events Randomized
Trial (FACET)[7] and Appropriate Blood Pressure Control in Diabetes
(ABCD) study,[8] have suggested that there may be differences in
outcome between the various anti-hypertensive drugs used; however,
this has not been substantiated in larger, more adequately powered
studies. Nevertheless, β blockers may be less suitable than other
agents for use in diabetic patients (see *β Blockers*, p. 179), although
their use is certainly not contra-indicated, and ACE inhibitors and
angiotensin receptor antagonists may confer benefits beyond blood
pressure reduction in terms of renoprotective effects (see below under
ACE inhibitors and *Angiotensin II receptor antagonists*).

> **Important:** The first-line choice of anti-hypertensive therapy
> in diabetic patients with hypertension is generally an ACE
> inhibitor or angiotensin receptor antagonist, unless there are
> compelling contra-indications for the use of these agents or
> compelling indications to use one of the other drugs.

ACE INHIBITORS

The ACE inhibitors are effective anti-hypertensive agents, with the
additional benefits of attenuating albuminuria and the progression of
renal disease beyond an effect on blood pressure alone. In addition,
ACE inhibition has been shown to reduce cardiovascular risk in
subjects with diabetes in both the Captopril Prevention Project
(CAPP) trial and Heart Outcomes Prevention Evaluation sub-study
MICRO HOPE. Furthermore, in the HOPE study, ACE inhibition was
shown to improve insulin resistance and prevent the development of

diabetes. The ACE inhibitors have also been shown to reduce the incidence of heart failure.

The ACE inhibitors should be the class of anti-hypertensive drug of first choice in diabetic patients with microalbuminuria or proteinuria.

> ⚠ **When starting therapy with an ACE inhibitor, caution should be exercised in patients with renovascular or peripheral vascular disease and also in those with a raised serum creatinine. Serum creatinine and electrolytes should be measured 1 week after initiating therapy with an ACE inhibitor and again following each increase in dosage.**

In situations where patients are unable to tolerate ACE inhibition due to cough or other side effects, angiotensin II receptor antagonists may be considered as alternative first-line therapy.

ANGIOTENSIN II RECEPTOR ANTAGONISTS

Angiotensin II receptor antagonists are recommended as initial therapy for diabetic patients with microalbuminuria who are unable to tolerate ACE inhibition. These agents are also suitable for use in patients with diabetes and coexisting proteinuria, with heart failure, post-myocardial infarction, and in renal insufficiency.

Three large trials have investigated the benefits of angiotensin II receptor blockade in subjects with diabetes and microalbuminuria or diabetic nephropathy:

- the Reduction of Endpoints in NIDDM with the Angiotensin II Antagonist Losartan (RENAAL) trial.[9]
- the Irbesartan Microalbuminuria Type 2 Diabetes in Hypertensive Patients (IRMA2) trial[10]
- the Irbesartan in Diabetic Nephropathy Trial.[11]

All have demonstrated benefit in reducing the progression of renal disease in patients with type 2 diabetes and hypertension. Because blood pressure reduction was similar in the placebo and angiotensin II receptor antagonist groups, renal protection appears, as with ACE inhibition, to be independent of blood pressure reduction.

The Losartan Intervention for Endpoint Reduction in Hypertension (LIFE) study reported the angiotensin II receptor antagonist losartan to be superior to the β blocker atenolol in reducing cardiovascular morbidity and mortality in a group of diabetic subjects with hypertension and left ventricular hypertrophy. Again, this effect appeared to be independent of blood pressure, because both treatment groups achieved the same reduction in blood pressure. In addition, losartan reduced the incidence of new diabetes by 25% compared with atenolol in the non-diabetic patients recruited to the LIFE study. Therefore, there is some suggestion that β blockers may be inferior to other drugs in the diabetic population.

β BLOCKERS

Despite the findings of the LIFE study and the fact that they may not be the first-line choice of therapy, β blockers can be effective anti-hypertensive agents in patients with diabetes. In the UKPDS, the β blocker atenolol was equally effective as the ACE inhibitor captopril in reducing stroke by 44% and diabetes-related death by 32%. Interestingly, the microvascular complications of diabetes were also reduced by 37%.

Data from sub-group analysis of other studies suggest that hypertensive individuals treated with β blockers have a greater risk of new-onset diabetes than control subjects or subjects receiving alternative anti-hypertensive therapy. Metabolic effects may vary with different B blockers. Indeed, the recent Glycemic Events in Diabetes Mellitus: Carvedilol-Metoprolol Comparison in Hypertensives (GEMINI) trial compared the effects of carvedilol and metoprolol on glycaemic control in 1235 patients with Type 2 diabetes mellitus and hypertension receiving renin-angiotensin system blockade; the trial showed that after a follow-up period of 35 weeks, carvedilol was superior to metoprolol in terms of insulin sensitivity, HbA1c level and progression to microalbuminuria in the cohort (Bakris GL, Fonseca V, Katholi RE, McGill JB, Messerli FH, Phillips RA, Raskin P, Wright JT Jr, Oakes R, Lukas MA, Anderson KM, Bell DS. Metabolic effects of carvedilol vs metoprolol in patients with type 2 diabetes mellitus and hypertension: a randomized controlled trial. JAMA 2004; Epub). Overall, there is good evidence of long-term benefit in terms of reducing cardiovascular disease in hypertensive patients with diabetes, and there is therefore no contra-indication to their use.

> **Important:** β Blockers should be particularly considered routinely in diabetic patients with ischaemic heart disease and angina, in whom they may be the drug of first choice, providing that the patient does not have microalbuminuria.

It should be remembered that non-selective β blockers may theoretically increase the risk of hypoglycaemia, although in practice this is rare. This effect is not a feature of selective β blockade, although treatment with selective β blockers may decrease the occurrence of the warning symptoms of hypoglycaemia.

CALCIUM CHANNEL BLOCKERS

Unlike β blockade and ACE inhibition, treatment with a calcium channel blocker has not been tested in a large cohort of patients with diabetes. However, in the Syst–Eur study there was a greater relative risk reduction in cardiovascular events in the 492 diabetic subjects treated with the long-acting calcium channel blocker nicardipine than in the non-diabetic individuals.

- Long-acting calcium channel blockers may be particularly useful in older diabetic patients with isolated systolic hypertension. Short-acting calcium channel blockers are, however, contra-indicated because these drugs may increase the risk of myocardial infarction.
- Because calcium channel blockers have some negative inotropic effect, they should not be used in diabetic patients with significant heart failure.
- Some calcium channel blockers also produce vasodilatation that can exacerbate postural hypertension, and these should be used with caution in diabetic individuals with autonomic neuropathy.
- As with β blockers, calcium channel blockers are likely to be particularly useful in patients with diabetes and angina.

THIAZIDE DIURETICS

As with the calcium channel blockers, the benefits of thiazide diuretics in terms of cardiovascular risk reduction have not been assessed in a large cohort of diabetic patients. However, thiazide diuretics are effective anti-hypertensive agents in patients with diabetes.

It has been suggested that the benefits of blood pressure reduction by thiazide diuretics may be offset by their metabolic side effects. However, adverse metabolic effects are observed only when these agents are used in large doses (50–200 mg of hydrochlorothiazide, over 5 mg of bendrofluazide), and these concerns have not been substantiated when lower doses that are effective anti-hypertensive agents have been used. Indeed, the 583 subjects with diabetes included in the Systolic Hypertension in the Elderly Program (SHEP) study, which used a diuretic-based regimen, obtained twice the absolute reduction in cardiovascular events compared with the non-diabetic group.

> **Important:** Diuretics are important as combination therapy in patients with diabetes, the majority of whom require more than a single agent for good control.

α BLOCKERS

α Blockers are effective anti-hypertensive agents and act via peripheral vasodilatation. They have not been adequately assessed as to their effect on reducing cardiovascular events in individuals with diabetes. However, they may have potential benefits in diabetes because they lower triglycerides and increase HDL cholesterol.

 α Blockers should be avoided in patients with severe autonomic dysfunction due to the high risk of severe postural hypotension.

BLOOD PRESSURE TREATMENT TARGETS IN DIABETES

The guidelines from the British Hypertension Society[12] and Joint National Committee (JNC 7)[13] state that treatment targets in most diabetic patients should be 130/80 mmHg or below. However, in diabetic patients with proteinuria the target blood pressure should probably be even lower.

The above blood pressure targets are difficult to achieve in many patients with type 2 diabetes, and combination therapy is often required. Indeed, 6 out of 10 subjects in the UKPDS needed two or more anti-hypertensive agents. The need for combination therapy is supported by data from 1372 patients with diabetes and hypertension, where the average number of anti-hypertensive agents to achieve a target blood pressure of 130/85 mmHg was 3.1.[14]

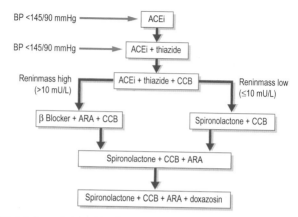

Fig. 4.4 Suggested algorithm for starting anti-hypertensive therapy in a patient with diabetes and hypertension. ACEi = angiotensin-converting enzyme inhibitor; CCB = calcuim channel blocker; ARA = angiotensin receptor antagonist.

> **Important:** Although usual practice is to start one anti-hypertensive agent at a time, if the starting blood pressure is well above targets, it may be better to introduce two agents within an initial short period of time, adding further agents later, as necessary.

Overall, the first-choice agent in the majority of diabetic patients is likely to be an ACE inhibitor or angiotensin receptor antagonist, followed by combination with a thiazide diuretic.

An example of an algorithm for starting therapy is shown in Fig. 4.4. However, based on the evidence to date, it would appear that improved cardiovascular outcomes as a result of pharmacological intervention appear to be associated mainly with consequent reduction in blood pressure rather than the agent used.

REFERENCES

1. Haffner S, Lehto S, Ronnemaa T, et al. Mortality from coronary heart disease in subjects with type 2 diabetes and in non-diabetic subjects with and without prior myocardial infarction. N Engl J Med 1998; 339: 229–234.

2. Hu FB, Stampfer MJ. Is type 2 diabetes mellitus a vascular condition? Arterioscler Thromb Vasc Biol 2003; 23(10): 1715–1716.

3. Gaede P, Vedel P, Larsen N, et al. Multifactorial intervention and cardiovascular disease in patients with type 2 diabetes. N Engl J Med 2003; 348(5): 383–393.

4. Malmberg K, Ryden L, Efendic S, et al. Randomized trial of insulin–glucose infusion followed by subcutaneous insulin treatment in diabetic patients with acute myocardial infarction (DIGAMI study): effects on mortality at 1 year. J Am Coll Cardiol 1995; 26(1): 57–65.

5. The UK Prospective Diabetes Study (UKPDS) Group. Tight blood pressure control and risk of macrovascular and microvascular complications in type II diabetes: UKPDS 38. Br Med J 1998; 317: 703–712.

6. Hansson L, Zanchetti A, Carruthers SG, et al. Effects of intensive blood-pressure lowering and low-dose aspirin in patients with hypertension: principal results of the Hypertension Optimal Treatment (HOT) randomised trial. HOT Study Group. Lancet 1998; 351(9118): 1755–1762.

7. Tatti P, Pahor M, Byington RP, et al. Outcome results of the Fosinopril Versus Amlodipine Cardiovascular Events Randomized Trial (FACET) in patients with hypertension and NIDDM. Diabetes Care 1998; 21(4): 597–603.

8. Estacio RO, Jeffers BW, Hiatt WR, et al. The effect of nisoldipine as compared with enalapril on cardiovascular outcomes in patients with non-insulin-dependent diabetes and hypertension. N Engl J Med 1998; 338(10): 645–652.

9. Brenner BM, Cooper ME, de Zeeuw D, et al. Effects of losartan on renal and cardiovascular outcomes in patients with type 2 diabetes and nephropathy. N Engl J Med 2001; 345(12): 861–869.

10. Lewis EJ, Hunsicker LG, Clarke WR, et al. Renoprotective effect of the angiotensin-receptor antagonist irbesartan in patients with nephropathy due to type 2 diabetes. N Engl J Med 2001; 345(12): 851–860.

11. Parving HH, Lehnert H, Brochner-Mortensen J, et al. The effect of irbesartan on the development of diabetic nephropathy in patients with type 2 diabetes. N Engl J Med 2001; 345(12): 870–878.

12. Williams B, Poulter NR, Brown MJ, et al. Guidelines for management of hypertension: report of the Fourth Working Party of the British Hypertension Society, 2004–BHS IV. J Hum Hypertens 2004; 18(3): 139–185.

13. Chobanian AV, Bakris GL, Black HR, et al. The seventh report of the Joint National Committee on Prevention, Detection, Evaluation, and Treatment of High Blood Pressure: the JNC 7 report. JAMA 2003; 289(19): 2560–2572.

14. Sowers JR, Epstein M, Frohlich ED. Diabetes, hypertension, and cardiovascular disease: an update. Hypertension 2001; 37(4): 1053–1059.

HYPERTENSION IN
THE ELDERLY

PREVALENCE AND TYPE OF HYPERTENSION

Hypertension in the elderly is a common problem. It affects more than half of over 60s if 160/100 mmHg or more is used as a definition, and more than 70% if the US Joint National Committee (JNC 7) criterion of 140/90 mmHg or more is employed (Fig. 4.5).[2]

By far the most common form of hypertension in older patients is isolated systolic hypertension. Indeed, isolated systolic hypertension accounts for more than 80% of hypertension in the over 60s (Fig. 4.6).[2–4] This pattern reflects the age-related widening of pulse pressure seen in almost all populations, which is a consequence of large artery stiffening, the result of fatigue fracture and disruption of

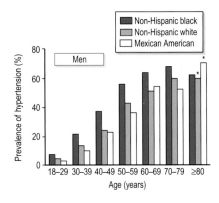

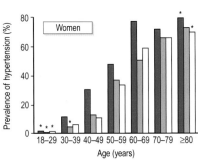

Fig. 4.5 Prevalence of hypertension by age in the USA (hypertension defined as blood pressure ≥ 140/90 mmHg). (From Burt et al 1995,[1] with permission of Lippincott, Williams and Wilkins.)

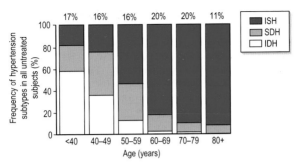

Fig. 4.6 Frequency of hypertension by type in the USA according to age: data from the National Health and Nutrition Examination Survey (NHANES III). (From Franklin et al 2001,[3] with permission of Lippincott, Williams and Wilkins.)

the elastic fibres within the arterial wall. Indeed, it is probable that everyone would develop isolated systolic hypertension should they live long enough.

Because the elderly are much more likely to develop hypertension than younger individuals, annual assessment of blood pressure in the over 60s seems sensible. It should be remembered that some automated sphygmomanometers may be unreliable in older individuals with stiffer arteries, and if in doubt a mercury device should be used.

PSEUDO-HYPERTENSION OF THE ELDERLY

Pseudo-hypertension refers to the situation where the brachial artery is markedly stiffened, often with calcification, and is thus resistant to compression by the sphygmomanometer cuff. Under these circumstances, cuff measurements invariably over-estimate true intra-arterial blood pressure. Unfortunately, the degree of discrepancy is highly variable, and it is often difficult to formulate an accurate management plan. Nevertheless, by virtue of increased large artery stiffness, such patients would appear to be at increased cardiovascular risk and thus stand to benefit from treatment, although titrating to target is almost impossible.

The clue to the presence of pseudo-hypertension is a positive Osler manoeuvre. In this test, a blood pressure cuff is inflated around the upper arm while palpating the radial pulse at the wrist. If the radial artery can still be clearly palpated when pulsation has ceased, pseudo-hypertension is likely.

RISK

As in younger age groups, there is a continuous relationship
between blood pressure and risk in older individuals (Fig. 4.7), and
there is no evidence of a J-shaped curve down to 115/75 mmHg.
Although the risk increment for each 20 mmHg rise in systolic blood
pressure in the over 80s is about half of that observed in middle-aged
individuals, the absolute differences in mortality are greater in older
age because the frequency of vascular events is so much higher. Thus
older patients stand to derive more benefit from therapy in absolute
terms.

Although originally considered to be benign and an inevitable
part of the ageing process, we now know that isolated systolic
hypertension considerably increases the risk of cardiovascular disease
and overall mortality (Fig. 4.8 and Table 4.1), and that treatment
brings considerable benefits.[8] Isolated systolic hypertension increases
the risk of stroke by around 60% and of coronary disease by around
40%. It is also a potent risk factor for heart failure.[9] Patients with so-
called 'borderline' isolated systolic hypertension (140–160 mmHg
and less than 90 mmHg) are also at increased cardiovascular risk, as
well as at increased risk of progression to established isolated systolic
hypertension.[9]

**TABLE 4.1 Risk of cardiovascular events by type of hypertension
in the Framingham Heart Study (36-year follow-up)**

| | Type of hypertension | | |
	Isolated diastolic	Isolated systolic	Combined
35–64 years			
Men	1.8*	2.4‡	2.7%‡
Women	1.2§	1.9†	2.2%‡
65–94 years			
Men	1.2*	1.9†	2.2%‡
Women	1.6‡	1.4†	1.6%‡

* Reference group consists of normotensive persons.
† $p < 0.05$; ‡ $p < 0.01$; § $p < 0.001$.
(From Kannel 2000,[7] with permission from Elsevier.)

BENEFITS OF THERAPY

The benefits of treating hypertension in the elderly have been well
documented in a number of different trials (see Table 4.2). This
applies to both elevated diastolic pressure with or without elevated

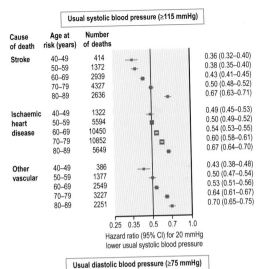

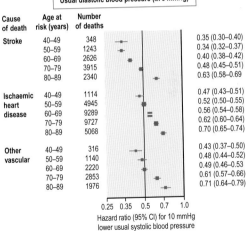

Fig. 4.7 The relationship between vascular mortality and blood pressure in different age groups: stroke, ischaemic heart disease, and other vascular mortality hazard ratios as a function of age for given differences in usual blood pressure. (From Lewington et al 2002,[5] with permission from Elsevier.)

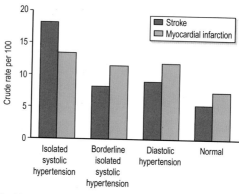

Fig. 4.8 Risks of isolated systolic hypertension: data from the Copenhagen Heart Study for 6621 untreated individuals aged over 50, followed up for 12 years on average. (From Nielsen et al 1999,[6] with permission.)

TABLE 4.2 Benefits of anti-hypertensive therapy in the elderly

Outcome measure	Reduction (%)	Number needed to treat
Cardiovascular morbidity and mortality	5.2	19
Cardiovascular mortality	2.0	50
Total mortality	1.7	63
(From Mulrow et al 2000[8])		

systolic pressure (Fig. 4.9) and elevated systolic pressure in isolation (Fig. 4.10). Indeed, a meta-analysis of eight trials with over 15 000 patients clearly demonstrated that cardiovascular events and total mortality are significantly reduced by therapy in patients with isolated systolic hypertension.[11] Moreover, the relative benefit from treatment in older patients is at least the same, if not greater, than that observed in younger individuals. Therefore, because the elderly are at higher risk of cardiovascular disease, they stand to gain a greater absolute risk reduction.

> **Important:** The available evidence suggests that all patients with sustained blood pressure greater than 160/100 mmHg should be treated, and this should be the first priority.

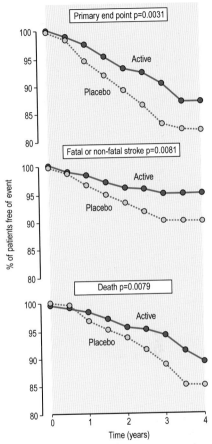

Fig. 4.9 Effect of anti-hypertensive treatment in older hypertensive patients: results of the Swedish Trial in Old Patients with Hypertension (STOP) in 70–84-year-olds treated with thiazides and β blockers or placebo. (From Dahlof et al 1991,[10] with permission from Elsevier.)

Individuals with pressures greater than 140/90 mmHg should receive therapy if their 10-year cardiovascular disease risk is over 20% or if there is evidence of end-organ damage, which includes coronary or cerebrovascular disease. This applies to patients with both essential hypertension and isolated systolic hypertension. Despite the clear

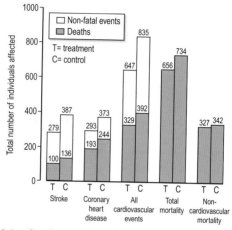

Fig. 4.10 Benefits of treatment in elderly individuals with isolated systolic hypertension: data from 15 693 patients during an average 3.8-year follow-up. The average blood pressure difference was 10/4 mmHg. T, treatment; C, control. (From Staessen et al 2000,[11] with permission from Elsevier.)

evidence supporting these recommendations, data from the UK and USA suggest that physicians have a bias against treating the elderly hypertensive patient.[12]

There is less evidence concerning the benefits of blood pressure reduction in the over 80s. However, around 15% of patients included in six major trials in this area were aged over 80 years, and a 1999 meta-analysis concluded that anti-hypertensive therapy is effective in reducing cardiovascular morbidity, but not mortality, in those aged over 80 years.[13] The Hypertension in the Very Elderly Trial (HYVET) will directly address this increasingly important issue, but until then it would seem appropriate to treat the very elderly who are otherwise well and have a reasonable quality of life.

TARGETS

The British Hypertension Society suggests that the target blood pressure is less than 140/85 mmHg for all patients, irrespective of age. However, this statement fails to recognize that isolated systolic hypertension, which is predominantly detected in the elderly, has a different pathophysiological basis to that of classical essential hypertension. Moreover, most physicians can testify to the difficulty of treating isolated systolic hypertension. Furthermore, data from three placebo-controlled trials indicate that a fall of just 10/4 mmHg is sufficient to reduce the risk of a cardiovascular event by a third.[14] Therefore, relatively modest reductions in blood pressure are certainly worthwhile. It may be more appropriate in clinical practice to aim for 140/85 mmHg in patients who start out at less than 160 mmHg, and to aim for a 20 mmHg reduction if the initial blood pressure is higher.

> **Important:** One thing to try to avoid in older patients is reducing diastolic pressure without altering systolic pressure (i.e. widening pulse pressure), which is often encountered in 'resistant' patients when potent vasodilator drugs are added, such as α blockers. In these circumstances, patients often feel unwell, perhaps due to a reduction in coronary artery perfusion, which occurs during diastole.

A post hoc analysis of the Systolic Hypertension in the Elderly Program (SHEP) trial suggests that lowering diastolic pressure below 70–60 mmHg may actually increase the risk of cardiovascular disease and stroke.[15]

SPECIFICS OF DRUG THERAPY IN THE ELDERLY

A wealth of evidence, including data from the Antihypertensive and Lipid-Lowering Treatment to Prevent Heart Attack Trial (ALLHAT), supports the view that thiazide diuretics should be first-line therapy for hypertension in the elderly (Fig. 4.11). Thiazides are, in general, well tolerated and effective when given at low doses (e.g. bendrofluazide 2.5 mg/day), and they are inexpensive. However, they are relatively ineffective if there is renal impairment (creatinine greater than 150 µmol/L) or concomitant use of non-steroidal anti-inflammatory drugs (see *Secondary hypertension*, p. 33). In such circumstances, long-acting dihydropyridine calcium channel blockers are a suitable alternative. However, short-acting dihydropyridines should not be used.

The Swedish Trial in Old Patients with Hypertension–2 (STOP–2) compared newer drugs (angiotensin-converting enzyme inhibitors and calcium channel blockers) with older drugs (thiazides and β blockers) in elderly anti-hypertensive subjects and found no real difference between agents (Fig. 4.12).[17] However, a 1998 meta-analysis implies

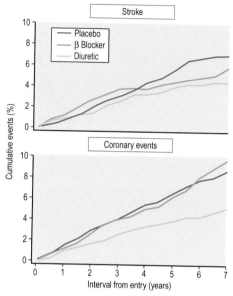

Fig. 4.11 Results of the MRC trial in hypertensive older adults: effect of thiazide, β blocker and placebo on stroke and coronary events. After adjustment for confounding variables, only thiazides significantly reduced both events. (From MRC Working Party 1992,[16] with permission of the BMJ Publishing Group.)

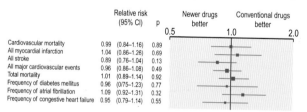

Fig. 4.12 Comparison of older and newer anti-hypertensive medication in older individuals: results of STOP–2 comparing thiazides and β blockers (conventional) with calcium channel blockers and angiotensin-converting enzyme inhibitors (new). There was no difference in any of the outcome measures. (From Hansson et al 1999,[17] with permission from Elsevier.)

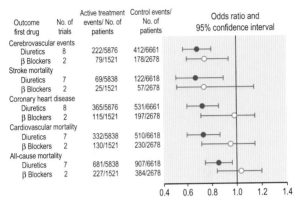

Outcome first drug	No. of trials	Active treatment events/ No. of patients	Control events/ No. of patients	Odds ratio and 95% confidence interval
Cerebrovascular events				
Diuretics	8	222/5876	412/6661	
β Blockers	2	79/1521	178/2678	
Stroke mortality				
Diuretics	7	69/5838	122/6618	
β Blockers	2	25/1521	57/2678	
Coronary heart disease				
Diuretics	8	365/5876	531/6661	
β Blockers	2	115/1521	197/2678	
Cardiovascular mortality				
Diuretics	7	332/5838	510/6618	
β Blockers	2	130/1521	230/2678	
All-cause mortality				
Diuretics	7	681/5838	907/6618	
β Blockers	2	227/1521	384/2678	

0.4 0.6 0.8 1.0 1.2 1.4

Fig. 4.13 Meta-analysis of thiazides versus β blockers in the elderly: the results suggest that β blockers have no significant effects on major outcome measures except for reducing cerebrovascular events. (From Messerli et al 1998,[18] with permission of JAMA.)

that some β blockers may be less efficacious than thiazides in the elderly (Fig. 4.13),[18] a finding that was also observed in the MRC trial in the elderly (Fig. 4.11), and in the LIFE study the outcome with atenolol-based therapy was less good than that with losartan-based therapy (see Fig. 3.9). For this reason, β blockers should probably not be used as first-line therapy in older hypertensive patients.

> **Important:** Potent vasodilators such as α blockers and minoxidil should be used with care in older patients with systolic hypertension, because these agents may induce postural hypotension and lower diastolic pressure, thus impoverishing coronary artery perfusion without having much impact on systolic blood pressure.

A useful alternative agent in patients resistant to standard combination therapy is the addition of a long-acting nitrate, for example isosorbide mononitrate modified release. Three separate trials indicate sustained blood pressure reduction with such agents in older hypertensive patents. However, hard outcome data are not available. Trial data indicate that many patients with systolic hypertension (around two-thirds) will require combination therapy to reach target. A practical algorithm is presented in Fig. 4.14.

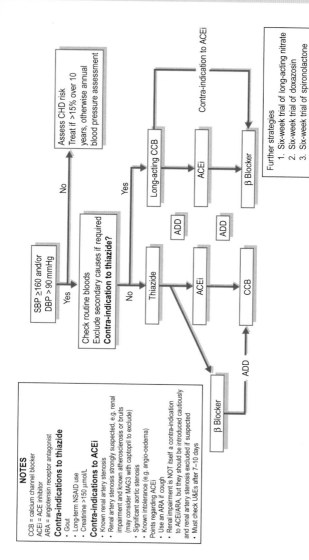

NOTES

CCB = calcium channel blocker
ACEi = ACE inhibitor
ARA = angiotensin receptor antagonist

Contra-indications to thiazide
- Gout
- Long-term NSAID use
- Creatinine >150 μmol/L

Contra-indications to ACEi
- Known renal artery stenosis
- Renal artery stenosis strongly suspected, e.g. renal impairment and known atherosclerosis or bruits (may consider MAG3 with captopril to exclude)
- Significant aortic stenosis
- Known intolerance (e.g. angio-oedema)

Points regarding ACEi
- Use an ARA if cough
- Renal impairment is NOT itself a contra-indication to ACEi/ARA, but they should be introduced cautiously and renal artery stenosis excluded if suspected
- Must check U&Es after 7–10 days

SBP ≥160 and/or DBP >90 mmHg

Yes → Check routine bloods / Exclude secondary causes if required / **Contra-indication to thiazide?**

No → Assess CHD risk / Treat if >15% over 10 years, otherwise annual blood pressure assessment

No → Thiazide → ACEi → CCB

ADD → β Blocker → ADD

Yes → Long-acting CCB → ACEi → β Blocker

Contra-indication to ACEi

ADD / ADD

Further strategies
1. Six-week trial of long-acting nitrate
2. Six-week trial of doxazosin
3. Six-week trial of spironolactone

Fig. 4.14 The treatment of hypertension in older patients.

PROBLEMS WITH BLOOD PRESSURE REDUCTION

In general, anti-hypertensive therapy is as well tolerated in the elderly as it is in younger patients. Indeed, withdrawal rates from placebo-controlled clinical trials are similar between placebo and active groups, and new and old drugs seem to be equally well tolerated. However, poly-pharmacy is an issue among older patients, and it can reduce patient compliance. The use of combination therapy and rational prescribing habits can help to minimize the number of drugs taken, as may the use of once-a-day formulations.

Some adverse effects, including postural hypotension and dizziness, can occur with the majority of anti-hypertensive medications, while others are drug-specific (e.g. bronchospasm with β blockers and gout with thiazides). However, the available evidence would suggest that adverse events are no more common in the elderly than in younger hypertensive patients. Moreover, several trials have failed to find any difference in symptom scores or quality of life measures between subjects randomized to active therapy and those taking placebo.[19] It is noteworthy that non-cardiovascular mortality is not significantly increased by therapy. Thus the concerns expressed by many physicians that any benefit from anti-hypertensive medication in the elderly will be offset by an excess of side effects, such as falls, seem largely unjustified. However, it may be appropriate to start with lower doses in the elderly and then to titrate against response and symptoms.

REFERENCES

1. Burt VL, Whelton P, Roccella EJ, et al. Prevalence of hypertension in the US adult population. Results of the Third National Health and Nutrition Examination Survey. Hypertension 1995; 25: 305–313.

2. Primatesta P, Brookes M, Poulter NR. Improved hypertension management and control: results from the health survey for England 1998. Hypertension 2001; 38(4): 827–832.

3. Franklin SS, Jacobs MJ, Wong ND, et al. Predominance of isolated systolic hypertension among middle-aged and elderly US hypertensives: analysis based on National Health and Nutrition Examination Survey (NHANES) III. Hypertension 2001; 37(3): 869–874.

4. Wilking SV, Belanger A, Kannel WB, et al. Determinants of isolated systolic hypertension. JAMA 1988; 260(23): 3451–3455.

5. Lewington S, Clarke R, Qizilbash N, et al. Prospective Studies Collaboration. Age-specific relevance of usual blood pressure to vascular mortality: a meta-analysis of individual data for one million adults in 61 prospective studies. Lancet 2002; 360: 1903–1913.

6. Nielsen WB, Vestbo J, Jensen GB, et al. Isolated systolic hypertension as a major risk factor for stroke and myocardial infarction and an unexploited source of cardiovascular prevention: a prospective population-based study. J Hum Hypertension 1999; 9: 175–180.

7. Kannel WB. Elevated systolic blood pressure as a cardiovascular risk factor. Am J Cardiol 2000; 85: 251.

8. Mulrow C, Lau J, Cornell J, et al. Pharmacotherapy for hypertension in the elderly (Cochrane Review). The Cochrane Library. Oxford: Update Software; 2000.

9. Sagie A, Larson MG, Levy D. The natural history of borderline systolic hypertension. N Engl J Med 1993; 329: 1912–1917.

10. Dahlof B, Lindholm LH, Hansson L, et al. Morbidity and mortality in the Swedish Trial in Old Patients with Hypertension (STOP–Hypertension). Lancet 1991; 338: 1281.

11. Staessen JA, Gasowski J, Wang JG, et al. Risks of untreated and treated isolated systolic hypertension in the elderly: meta-analysis of outcome trials. Lancet 2000; 355(9207): 865–872.

12. Dickerson JEC, Brown MJ. Influence of age on general practitioners' definition and treatment of hypertension. Br Med J 1995; 310: 574.

13. Gueyffier F, Bulpitt C, Boissel JP, et al. Antihypertensive drugs in very old people: a subgroup meta-analysis of randomised controlled trials. INDANA Group. Lancet 1999; 353(9155): 793–796.

14. Staessen JA, Gasowski J, Wang JG, et al. Risks of untreated and treated isolated systolic hypertension in the elderly: meta-analysis of outcome trials. Lancet 2000; 355(9207): 865–872.

15. Somes GW, Pahor M, Shorr RI, et al. The role of diastolic blood pressure when treating isolated systolic hypertension. Arch Intern Med 1999; 159(17): 2004–2009.

16. MRC Working Party. Medical Research Council trial of treatment of hypertension in older adults: principal results. Br Med J 1992; 304: 405–412.

17. Hansson L, Lindholm LH, Ekbom T, et al. Randomised trial of old and new antihypertensive drugs in elderly patients: cardiovascular mortality and morbidity in the Swedish Trial in Old Patients with Hypertension–2 study. Lancet 1999; 354(9192): 1751–1756.

18. Messerli FH, Grossman E, Goldbourt U. Are beta-blockers efficacious as first-line therapy for hypertension in the elderly? A systematic review. JAMA 1998; 279(23): 1903–1907.

19. O'Donnell CJ, Ridker PM, Glynn RJ, et al. Hypertension and borderline isolated systolic hypertension increase risks of cardiovascular disease and mortality in male physicians. Circulation 1997; 95(5): 1132–1137.

HYPERTENSION IN THE OBESE PATIENT

Many patients with hypertension are overweight; however, some are clinically obese (body mass index, BMI, over 30 kg/m^2). There are special considerations in both the diagnosis and management of hypertension in the obese patient.

BLOOD PRESSURE MEASUREMENT IN THE OBESE PATIENT

As in the non-obese patient, blood pressure measurements should be made using an appropriately sized cuff, with the bladder encircling at least two-thirds of the upper arm circumference (see Fig. 2.4, p. 76). Measurements made in an obese arm using a standard-sized blood pressure cuff will over-estimate the true blood pressure. Patients with a significant amount of subcutaneous fat tissue in the upper arm may find inflation of a blood pressure cuff particularly uncomfortable and even painful. Also, if the upper arms of an obese patient are tending towards a conical shape, placement of a cuff around the arm can be very difficult. In both of these instances, wrist cuff blood pressure measurements using a specially designed measuring device may be a suitable alternative.

MANAGEMENT OF HYPERTENSION IN THE OBESE PATIENT

One of the primary goals in the management of hypertension in the obese patient must be weight reduction through a combination of diet, healthy eating and exercise. It may be appropriate to involve a dietician or to discuss whether the patient would benefit from joining a club to help with weight loss.

Important: It should be emphasized that calorific restriction is necessary for initial weight loss; however, unless a healthy eating pattern is adopted long term, it will be difficult to maintain any weight loss achieved.

A good incentive to encourage weight loss is that it may be possible to avoid the use of anti-hypertensive medication or to reduce the number of medications required if the patient loses a reasonably substantial amount of weight. Also, weight loss:

- will improve patients' overall cardiovascular risk and risk of diabetes
- may improve their lipid profile
- may improve their body image and general well-being.

Important: Alcohol is a high calorific source, and obese patients should be encouraged to limit their alcohol intake, again producing weight loss but also with blood pressure-lowering effects in its own right.

In addition to aiding weight loss, regular exercise has synergistic blood pressure-lowering effects; therefore patients should be encouraged to incorporate more exercise into their lives. For severely obese people this may be difficult. One approach might be to initially introduce simple exercise as part of the daily routine, for example:

- using stairs instead of lifts
- getting off buses one stop earlier and walking the remainder of the journey
- parking further away from work and walking.

Gradually, as patients become more accustomed to exercise, this routine can be built up to include some light exercise, which will become easier as weight loss continues. In some areas, systems are in place whereby patients can be referred directly to a local gym by their doctor, in order to start a weight reduction programme.

In the case of severe obesity, it may be appropriate to refer the patient to a specialist in the treatment of obesity for further advice. In patients with a BMI greater than 30 kg/m^2 who have failed to achieve reasonable weight loss despite at least 3 months' trial of the above measures, some benefit may be gained from specific drug therapy to target obesity. These drugs should be used only as an adjunct to lifestyle measures and should be prescribed and monitored by specialists in the field.

DRUG THERAPY FOR OBESITY

Orlistat is a lipase inhibitor that reduces the absorption of dietary fat. By inhibiting fat absorption it causes significant steatorrhoea, which often causes patients to reduce the amount of fat in their diets to avoid this unpleasant side effect. It may be necessary to supplement the diet with fat-soluble vitamins, particularly vitamin D, because their absorption may be impaired while on treatment. Guidelines recommend that the use of orlistat should usually be limited to up to 1 year and certainly not for more than 2 years. It is not licensed for use in children.

An alternative anti-obesity drug is sibutramine. This is a centrally acting appetite suppressant that inhibits serotonin and noradrenaline reuptake. Again, its use should be carefully monitored. It can cause worsening of hypertension and tachycardia.

DRUG THERAPY FOR HYPERTENSION IN THE OBESE PATIENT

Obese patients with hypertension tend to have a higher sympathetic drive than non-obese patients. However, the choice of drug therapy to treat hypertension in the obese patient is not significantly different to that in the non-obese. In younger patients, treatment should commence with either an angiotensin-converting enzyme inhibitor or a β blocker, and in older patients with a thiazide diuretic or calcium channel blocker. There may be a case for reviewing the drug doses used because obese patients may require a slightly higher dose than people of much lower body weight.

> **Important:** It is important to carefully screen obese patients for glucose intolerance or frank diabetes mellitus, because these conditions are more common with increasing BMI values.

HYPERTENSION IN PREGNANCY

Hypertension is a feature of around 5–10% of pregnancies and is the second commonest cause of maternal death after thromboembolic disease. Hypertensive disease of pregnancy also carries significant morbidity and mortality risk for the fetus.

> **Important:** Guidelines regarding the level of blood pressure that should be treated in pregnancy vary; however, in general most physicians would agree that treatment should be considered for any woman with blood pressure consistently higher than 140/90 mmHg and drug therapy should almost definitely be started if the blood pressure is higher than 160/100 mmHg.

The final decision on whether or not to start drug therapy will depend on:

- the degree of hypertension
- the stage of pregnancy
- a discussion with the patient of the risks versus the benefits of treatment.

The target for blood pressure lowering in pregnancy is usually around 140/90 mmHg. There is no benefit to be gained from lowering the blood pressure further.

In pregnant women, it can be difficult to hear the fourth phase of Korotkoff sounds (continuous muffling) when measuring diastolic blood pressure using a mercury sphygmomanometer. Therefore the fifth phase (disappearance of sound) should be recorded as a measure of diastolic pressure. In a few women the sound fails to disappear, and in these women the fourth Korotkoff sound may be taken as the diastolic pressure, but this should be noted carefully in the records.

NORMAL BLOOD PRESSURE CHANGES IN PREGNANCY

During normal pregnancy, various circulatory changes take place due to the actions of sex hormones and the effects of the placenta on regional blood flow. Early in pregnancy, there is a reduction in peripheral vascular resistance. Other haemodynamic changes occurring later in pregnancy include increased circulating plasma volume, increased cardiac output, increased renal blood flow, and increased glomerular filtration rate.

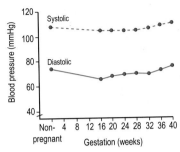

Fig. 4.15 Normal changes in blood pressure during pregnancy: blood pressure decreases during the late first and second trimesters before increasing in later pregnancy.

- Overall, blood pressure in the first trimester tends to be similar to pre-conception blood pressure.
- In the second trimester, there tends to be a reduction in blood pressure of a few mmHg.
- In the third trimester, blood pressure rises again; this is the trimester in which there is the greatest risk of the development of high blood pressure or even pre-eclampsia (Fig. 4.15).

The blood pressure changes described above also occur in women who are hypertensive before the time of conception, such that the blood pressure will again be lowest in the second trimester.

Important: In women who are hypertensive before conception, adjustment of anti-hypertensive therapy during the second trimester may be necessary to compensate for normal physiological changes.

DEFINITION OF HYPERTENSION IN PREGNANCY

The definition of hypertension in pregnancy is complex, because it includes:

- pre-existing hypertension
- hypertension that develops during pregnancy
- pre-eclampsia and eclampsia.

The last of these are conditions with their own particular features, one of which is hypertension. It is therefore simplest to classify the condition under the sub-headings shown in Box 4.5. The different types of hypertension in pregnancy are discussed in more detail below.

Box 4.5 Classification of hypertension in pregnancy

Chronic (pre-existing) hypertension
Systolic blood pressure ≥ 140 mmHg and/or diastolic blood pressure ≥ 90 mmHg before the 20th week of pregnancy.
May be associated with proteinuria and usually persists post partum.

Pregnancy-induced (gestational) hypertension
Systolic blood pressure ≥ 140 mmHg and/or diastolic blood pressure ≥ 90 mmHg developing after the 20th week of pregnancy *or* ≥ 30/15-mmHg rise in blood pressure compared with first-trimester or pre-conception blood pressure, in the absence of pre-eclampsia.
Returns to normal post partum.

Pre-eclampsia
Multisystem disorder usually occurring in the third trimester of pregnancy. Hypertension* with proteinuria > 300 mg/24 hours.
Marked oedema often occurs in pre-eclampsia but no longer forms part of the definition of the disorder.

Pre-eclampsia superimposed on chronic hypertension
New proteinuria, sudden increases in blood pressure or proteinuria, thrombocytopenia, or increases in hepatocellular enzymes in pregnancy in patients with chronic hypertension.

*A ≥ 15-mmHg rise in diastolic blood pressure or ≥ 25 mmHg in systolic blood pressure from early pregnancy *or* a single diastolic blood pressure reading of ≥ 110 mmHg *or* two readings 4 hours apart of ≥ 90 mmHg.

PRE-ECLAMPSIA

 Pre-eclampsia is a serious condition that must be identified early and treated appropriately to prevent morbidity and mortality for the mother and fetus.

Screening for the development of pre-eclampsia is one of the most important goals of antenatal visits, particularly in the third trimester of pregnancy, when blood pressure measurements and urinalysis should be performed at least fortnightly. Although pre-eclampsia is most common in the third trimester, it can also develop up to 1 week following delivery of the fetus. Therefore blood pressure should also be monitored around the time of and after delivery.

The main maternal risks of pre-eclampsia are of:

- stroke
- cardiac arrhythmias
- ischaemic heart disease
- acute renal failure.

If not treated adequately, pre-eclampsia may progress to eclampsia, a condition in which the mother suffers generalized tonic–clonic seizures and both mother and fetus are at very high risk of death. Pre-eclampsia is also thought to cause impaired placentation leading to intra-uterine growth retardation or even fetal death. If early delivery is required due to pre-eclampsia, prematurity is also an important issue.

Pre-eclampsia is a multisystem disease, the mechanisms of which are not yet fully understood. There may be some genetic predisposition and there are several other risk factors for the development of the condition (Box 4.6). Of note, women with chronic (pre-existing) hypertension are at increased risk of developing pre-eclampsia. Widespread vascular dysfunction occurs in pre-eclampsia, with a reduction in nitric oxide and prostacyclin production and an increase in thromboxane A2 production. This leads to vasospasm and vascular occlusion causing ischaemia of organs.

- The features of pre-eclampsia include a rise in blood pressure associated with proteinuria of over 300 mg/24 hours.
- Other features include oedema, particularly of the face and hands, which is non-dependent in nature; coagulation abnormalities; and elevation of hepatocellular enzymes.

Box 4.6 Risk factors for pre-eclampsia

First pregnancy
Pre-eclampsia in previous pregnancy
Younger (age < 20 years) or older (age > 35 years) at
   time of pregnancy
Short stature
Family history of pre-eclampsia or eclampsia
Previous hypertension
Multiple pregnancy (i.e. twins, triplets, etc.)
Change of partner since previous pregnancy
Migraine
Underweight
Raynaud's disease
Systemic lupus erythematosus
Hydatidiform mole

- Serum urate levels usually rise due to reduced excretion of urate at the proximal tubule of the kidney.
- Severe vasospasm associated with high blood pressure and coagulation abnormalities may lead to ischaemic or haemorrhagic stroke, myocardial infarction or renal failure.
- The haemolysis, elevated liver enzymes and low platelets (HELLP) syndrome is at the more severe end of the spectrum of pre-eclampsia.

If pre-eclampsia is diagnosed, the woman should be admitted to hospital and confined to bed rest. Anti-hypertensive agents that are safe in pregnancy may be used to lower the blood pressure, typically labetalol or methyldopa (see *Drug therapy for hypertension in pregnancy*, p. 211). The following should be monitored regularly:

- blood pressure
- proteinuria
- fetal cardiotocograph
- full blood count
- urea and electrolytes
- liver function tests
- urate levels.

While it may be possible to control the blood pressure with anti-hypertensive therapy, the only definitive cure for pre-eclampsia is delivery of the fetus, and timing of this will depend on:

- the condition of the mother
- the degree of severity of pre-eclampsia
- whether there are any signs of fetal distress.

Where premature delivery is unavoidable, it may be possible to give corticosteroids to the mother for 24 hours before delivery to mature the fetal lungs and reduce the risk of respiratory distress syndrome in the baby.

> **⚠ If eclampsia develops, seizures should be treated with intravenous magnesium sulphate and phenytoin if required; blood pressure should be controlled using intravenous labetalol, glyceryl trinitrate, sodium nitroprusside or hydralazine; and immediate delivery of the fetus should be carried out.**

All women who have suffered from pre-eclampsia or eclampsia should be followed up for a number of weeks to ensure that their blood pressure returns to normal post partum. Anti-hypertensive therapy should be withdrawn gradually, and by 6 weeks post partum it should be possible to be free of anti-hypertensive therapy, unless there is underlying chronic hypertension.

Although the risk of pre-eclampsia is highest with the first pregnancy, women who have suffered pre-eclampsia with a previous pregnancy are at increased risk of pre-eclampsia in future pregnancies. Also, women with pre-eclampsia have an increased risk of developing chronic hypertension later in life, which is estimated at 15% at 2 years.

OTHER FORMS OF HYPERTENSION IN PREGNANCY

CHRONIC (PRE-EXISTING) HYPERTENSION

The management of chronic hypertension begins even before conception.

- Any woman of childbearing age who requires drug therapy for hypertension should be counselled about contraception and whether she has any plans to become pregnant in the future.
- If anti-hypertensive therapy is definitely required, it is preferable to choose a regimen that would be safe in pregnancy.

If the hypertension is relatively mild, it may be possible to discontinue any medication prior to conception, in the knowledge that blood pressure levels tend to stay relatively constant during the first trimester and fall during the second trimester, tending to rise again only during the third trimester, when treatment can be restarted if necessary. This has the advantage of avoiding the risk of fetal malformation due to drugs in the early part of pregnancy while organogenesis is taking place. Even if a drug that is considered to be safe is given during early pregnancy, if a fetal malformation occurs (which happens anyway in around 3% of pregnancies), the woman (and physician) may be left with doubt over whether or not the drug was responsible.

PREGNANCY-INDUCED (GESTATIONAL) HYPERTENSION

Pregnancy-induced hypertension usually manifests in the third trimester but may occur at any time after 20 weeks of gestation. It is differentiated from pre-eclampsia by the presence of an elevated blood pressure without the other features of pre-eclampsia.

- If anti-hypertensive therapy is considered necessary, one of the drugs considered to be safe in pregnancy (see *Drug therapy for hypertension in pregnancy* below) should be given at the lowest dose necessary to control the blood pressure.
- The patient should be monitored regularly and screened for the development of pre-eclampsia.

By definition, pregnancy-induced hypertension should resolve by 6 weeks post partum. Anti-hypertensive therapy can therefore be weaned off during the first few weeks following delivery. If the hypertension persists after the sixth week post partum, it is not pregnancy-induced hypertension and is better classified as chronic hypertension, in which case the need for continuing anti-hypertensive therapy should be considered.

A RARE FORM OF HYPERTENSION IN PREGNANCY

A very rare form of severe hypertension in pregnancy is due to a mutation causing a single amino acid substitution in the mineralocorticoid receptor,[1] which causes constitutive receptor activation and alters receptor sensitivity such that progesterone and certain other steroids that normally antagonize the receptor now activate it, leading to salt and water retention and hypertension. This mutation causes early-onset hypertension that may show cyclical variation with the menstrual cycle and which is exacerbated greatly in early pregnancy due to the high levels of progesterone.

DRUG THERAPY FOR HYPERTENSION IN PREGNANCY

Most drugs are not licensed for use in pregnancy; therefore the choice of anti-hypertensive therapy is limited to those that are thought to be safe. It is best to avoid all drugs in the first trimester if possible.

> ⚠ **Some anti-hypertensive agents are absolutely contra-indicated in pregnancy due to fetotoxicity; for example, angiotensin-converting enzyme inhibitors cause serious renal toxicity in the fetus.**

The most commonly used first-choice anti-hypertensive agents in pregnancy are:

- the combined α and β blocker labetalol *or*
- the centrally acting agent methyldopa.

Both of these agents have been used in pregnancy for many years and are considered to be safe. Labetalol is contra-indicated in asthma and methyldopa may cause side effects including depression. Other agents that may be used if necessary in late pregnancy include the calcium channel blocker nifedipine (modified release), which is thought to be safe, and β blockers such as atenolol or bisoprolol, although there is some evidence to suggest that β blockers may retard fetal growth.

> **Important:** The decision to use any of these agents during pregnancy must be based on an analysis of the benefits to the mother (and fetus) versus the risks to the fetus (and mother), and the decision to treat should be made by a specialist.

Table 4.3 lists some anti-hypertensive agents and whether they can be used safely in pregnancy. In the UK, up-to-date information on prescribing in pregnancy is available in publications such as the British National Formulary, and further detailed information on drugs

TABLE 4.3 Use of anti-hypertensive drugs in pregnancy

Anti-hypertensive drug or class	Status in pregnancy
β Blockers	Labetalol (combined α and β blocker) thought to be safe. May cause mild intra-uterine growth retardation. Avoid in asthmatics. Other β blockers (e.g. atenolol, bisoprolol). May cause intra-uterine growth retardation, neonatal bradycardia and hypoglycaemia, prolonged labour. Use by specialist only. Avoid in asthmatic patients. Avoid in early pregnancy. Probably safe in third trimester.
Methyldopa	Thought to be safe. May cause depression, drowsiness, diarrhoea. Avoid if history of depression.
Calcium channel blockers	Nifedipine modified release. Limited data but thought to be safe.
Angiotensin-converting enzyme inhibitors	*Contra-indicated.* If given in second or third trimester, may cause neonatal renal failure, oligohydramnios, structural defects, pulmonary hypoplasia, intra-uterine death. No evidence of increased birth defects if given in first trimester.
Angiotensin receptor antagonists	*Contra-indicated.* Limited data in humans but animal data suggest serious fetotoxicity.
Thiazide diuretics	*Avoid if possible.* May interfere with plasma volume expansion.

in pregnancy is available from the National Teratology Information Service (telephone 0191 232 1525). For many of the newer anti-hypertensive agents, limited data exist on whether or not they are safe in pregnancy, and these are therefore best avoided in favour of the more established drugs, which have a body of evidence suggesting their effects in pregnancy.

REFERENCE

1. Geller DS, Farhi A, Pinkerton N, et al. Activating mineralocorticoid receptor mutation in hypertension exacerbated by pregnancy. Science 2000; 289(5476): 119–123.

ETHNIC AND RACIAL DIFFERENCES

RESPONSE TO THERAPY

In general, Afro-Caribbean populations tend to have a higher prevalence of hypertension than white people. In addition, the onset of hypertension in these populations tends to be at an earlier age and they have a higher risk of complications, particularly of stroke and hypertensive renal disease. In fact, the prevalence of hypertensive renal disease is 17.7 times higher in black patients than in white patients. Even in young hypertensive patients, black people show a higher prevalence of microalbuminuria than white patients. Black patients also show different 24-hour blood pressure profiles, with a higher rate of nocturnal 'non-dippers' (see *Measurement of blood pressure*, p. 73). This higher nocturnal blood pressure may be partly responsible for the increase in microalbuminuria.

Black people with hypertension tend to have a low-renin, volume-expanded form of hypertension. They are generally more salt-sensitive than white people, and therefore reductions in dietary salt intake in black people have more effect in terms of blood pressure lowering. The altered sodium handling may be partly related to polymorphisms of the α-adducin gene that are more common in the black populations.

In terms of response to anti-hypertensive therapy, black people tend to respond better to diuretics and calcium channel blockers than to drugs acting directly against the renin–angiotensin system such as angiotensin-converting enzyme (ACE) inhibitors and β blockers. In this aspect, they behave similarly to elderly white patients who also have a low-renin form of hypertension.

> **Important:** The first-choice anti-hypertensive therapy for the majority of black patients will be either a thiazide diuretic or a calcium channel blocker. ACE inhibitors or β blockers may have more effect in these patients once their renin–angiotensin system is activated by concurrent therapy with diuretics.

Racial differences in the β_2-adrenoceptor polymorphism may account for some of the difference in response to some of the more non-selective β blockers. Indeed, a study looking at the highly β_1-selective β blocker bisoprolol showed little difference in response rates between black and white patients. Racial differences in the ACE genotype may also influence the response to ACE inhibitor therapy.

RISK OF MALIGNANT HYPERTENSION

Black Africans are at an increased risk of malignant hypertension than are white people. A number of factors may contribute to this risk, including:

- genetic and environmental differences
- racial differences in renal physiology
- inadequate treatment of hypertension in some socio-economic groups
- the higher prevalence of end-stage renal disease.

Black Africans are at particular risk of cerebral haemorrhage as a feature of malignant hypertension. The treatment of acute episodes of malignant hypertension does not differ between black and white people; however, the long-term maintenance therapy may differ as described earlier, being based on thiazide diuretic or calcium channel blocker therapy.

CHILDREN AND ADOLESCENTS

BLOOD PRESSURE MEASUREMENT

Blood pressure is measured in children in a similar way to in adults using either mercury sphygmomanometry, or aneroid or automated devices. Small cuffs are available to fit infants and children.

- The bladder of the cuff should encompass 80–100% of the arm.
- The width of the cuff should be 40% of the upper arm circumference.

Blood pressure in children rises with age, and with increasing weight and height. The closest correlation is with height, and for this reason blood pressure measurements in children are usually checked against a centile chart relating blood pressure to height. Blood pressure measurements lying:

- below the 90th centile for height are regarded as normal
- between the 90th and 95th centile are high normal
- on or above the 95th centile are abnormal.

As for adults, at least three readings should be taken on separate occasions before diagnosing hypertension.

Hypertension is very rare in infants and remains rare in children, increasing in prevalence in older adolescents. Most cases of hypertension in children are secondary to underlying causes (see further and also *Secondary hypertension*, p. 33). Essential hypertension becomes more common in adolescents.

There is no evidence for benefit of screening children for hypertension. It is recommended that blood pressure should be measured as part of the assessment of any ill child, and it should also be regularly assessed if they have any risk factors such as:

- bladder, kidney or ureteric disease
- diabetes mellitus
- a previous history of high blood pressure readings
- a family history of hypertension at a young age.

There is no consensus on the benefits of treating hypertension in children and adolescents; however, there is evidence from longitudinal studies that children who are hypertensive have a four times higher risk of having hypertension as adults.

SECONDARY HYPERTENSION

Most hypertension in infants and young children is secondary to an underlying disease. The commonest disorders causing secondary hypertension in children include:

- renal parenchymal disease such as glomerulonephritis
- renovascular disease
- coarctation of the aorta
- reflux nephropathy
- endocrine disorders
- neoplasms.

> **Important:** It should be remembered that excessive consumption of liquorice causes hypertension due to its aldosterone-like actions on sodium transport in the kidney. This possibility can be excluded by taking a detailed history and the condition responds to cessation of liquorice intake.

CHOICE OF ANTI-HYPERTENSIVE THERAPY

If there is an underlying disorder causing the hypertension, this should be treated appropriately. However, some children will require regular anti-hypertensive therapy to control their blood pressure and to reduce damage to the end organs.

There is no evidence that any one group of drugs is better than the others in treating children. Some of the agents used in the treatment of adult hypertension are not licensed for use in children.

> **Important:** Overall, angiotensin-converting enzyme inhibitors, calcium channel blockers, diuretics and β blockers are generally considered to be safe and effective in children with hypertension. Drug doses are determined by weight of the child, and some agents are available as elixirs, aiding palatability.

For the treatment of hypertensive emergencies in children, a variety of options exist including:

- intravenous labetalol
- sodium nitroprusside
- nicardipine.

PSEUDO-HYPERTENSION OF YOUTH

Pseudo-hypertension of youth is a condition that has been described in young, fit, tall men from adolescence up to the age of 30 years.[1,2] These patients have elevated systolic blood pressure when measured at the arm in the conventional way. However, their aortic systolic blood pressures are relatively normal. This condition is thought to be due to an exaggeration of the normal amplification of the blood pressure from the aorta to the arm. Diastolic and mean arterial pressures are usually normal. Some of these patients have unusually distensible arteries.

It is not known whether pseudo-hypertension of youth is a benign condition or whether these people are at higher risk of later hypertension and cardiovascular disease. Further investigation of this condition is required to answer this question, and at present any young patient with high blood pressure should be referred to specialists for assessment.

REFERENCES

1. O'Rourke M, Vlachopoulos C, Graham RM. Spurious systolic hypertension in youth. Vasc Med 2000; 5: 141–145.
2. Mahmud A, Feely J. Spurious systolic hypertension of youth: fit young men with elastic arteries. Am J Hypertens 2003; 16(3): 229–232.

CHAPTER 5

FREQUENTLY ASKED QUESTIONS IN HYPERTENSION

WHAT IS HYPERTENSION?

Hypertension is simply raised or high blood pressure. Because blood pressure varies widely within a population and also varies from minute to minute, it is difficult to give a precise definition of hypertension. However, most authorities would suggest that a *sustained* elevation of blood pressure above 140/90 mmHg can be termed *hypertension*. Hypertension does not always require treatment but should always be investigated further once identified.

WHAT CAUSES HYPERTENSION?

In the vast majority of patients, no underlying cause is ever found for hypertension, and thus it is termed *essential hypertension*. In a small number of patients (5–10%) an underlying cause can be identified, and this offers the possibility of a cure for these patients. A number of different causes have been described, ranging from disorders of the adrenal glands and kidneys to drugs such as the oral contraceptive pill (see *Secondary hypertension*, p. 33).

In physiological terms, in the majority of patients, essential hypertension is due to an increased resistance to blood flow, which usually results from changes in the very small arteries. However, in older patients, essential hypertension usually comes about due to a hardening or stiffening of the larger arteries.

WHAT ARE THE RISKS OF HYPERTENSION?

In the long term, hypertension is associated with a number of adverse consequences. These include left ventricular hypertrophy and ultimately heart failure, renal damage, retinopathy, and structural functional changes in the arterial tree. Hypertension is an important risk factor for the development of atherosclerosis, which may manifest as cerebrovascular disease, coronary artery disease or peripheral vascular disease. It also increases the risk of haemorrhagic stroke and sub-arachnoid haemorrhage.

The vast majority of patients with hypertension are asymptomatic. Although headache is often attributed to hypertension, this is rare; previous studies have found that headache is no more common in hypertensive people than in the general population. However, in the minority of patients with secondary hypertension, symptoms may be elicited due to the presence of the underlying condition, such as palpitations or heart failure in individuals with phaeochromocytoma, or muscle weakness in those with Conn's syndrome. Symptoms are common in patients with malignant hypertension, and range from headaches to confusion, loss of consciousness, and seizures.

DOES HYPERTENSION RUN IN FAMILIES?

Hypertension is more common in individuals with a family history of hypertension. Certain rare monogenic forms of hypertension, such as Gordon's syndrome and glucocorticoid-remediable aldosteronism, show clear patterns of inheritance within individual families. However, in essential hypertension a genetic linkage is much weaker (but certainly present), and as yet the genes underlying this remain to be identified; essential hypertension most likely represents the inter-play between a number of genes with relatively small blood pressure-raising effects and environmental stimuli and stresses.

WHAT IS WHITE COAT HYPERTENSION?

White coat hypertension simply refers to the situation in which a patient's blood pressure is raised in the setting of clinic blood pressure measurements (e.g. a general practitioner's surgery) but normal at other times. This is usually detected by the use of ambulatory blood pressure monitoring or home blood pressure monitoring, but the literature is split as to whether such patients are at higher risk of developing subsequent sustained hypertension or whether they are at increased risk of cardiovascular disease (see p. 19).

WHICH LIFESTYLE CHANGES AFFECT THE REDUCTION IN BLOOD PRESSURE?

Changes in lifestyle can have modest effects on blood pressure reduction (see *Lifestyle factors and relationship with hypertension*, p. 27, and *Lifestyle measures*, p. 97). Weight loss—especially when combined with exercise, exercise itself, salt reduction, and reduction in alcohol intake—has been shown to be effective. Reduction in caffeine intake can have at best a small effect (1–2 mmHg), but the jury is still out as to whether stress–relaxation therapies are effective.

DOES STRESS MAKE HYPERTENSION WORSE?

Although it has been suggested that essential hypertension in its early phases may be due to over-activity of the sympathetic nervous system, the link between stress and hypertension is still unclear. Stress may play a role, but it is certainly not the primary problem in the vast majority of patients with essential hypertension. Moreover, no randomized, appropriately controlled, trial has ever shown that stress reduction techniques lead to a fall in blood pressure.

CAN HIGH BLOOD PRESSURE BE CURED?

In patients with secondary hypertension, appropriate treatment of the underlying cause may result in a cure. However, this is not necessarily the case, and even in patients with conditions such as Conn's disease—in whom a biochemical cure is achieved following surgical removal of the aldosterone-secreting adenoma—hypertension can persist, although it is often much easier to manage.

In patients with essential hypertension, even aggressive anti-hypertensive therapy fails to bring about a cure. Therefore, as long as the correct diagnosis was made at the outset, essential hypertension is at present incurable and management concentrates on achieving good blood pressure control. Patients should be told at the outset that they are likely to require lifelong therapy.

WHICH PATIENTS ARE LIKELY TO HAVE SECONDARY HYPERTENSION?

Secondary hypertension is more likely in people with accelerated or malignant hypertension, and in young patients with early-onset hypertension. Clearly, signs and symptoms may also point to secondary hypertension (see *Secondary hypertension*, p. 33).

WHEN SHOULD DRUG TREATMENT BE STARTED IN HYPERTENSION?

All patients with a sustained blood pressure elevation over 160/100 mmHg should receive therapy. Those with blood pressure over 140/90 mmHg with a 10-year cardiovascular disease risk greater than 20%, evidence of end-organ damage, diabetes mellitus, or previous cardiovascular disease should also be considered for therapy.

WHICH DRUG IS THE FIRST CHOICE FOR HYPERTENSION?

Guidance from the British Hypertension Society suggests that first-line therapy should be with:

- an angiotensin-converting enzyme (ACE) inhibitor or a β blocker in younger patients
- a thiazide or a calcium channel blocker in older patients.

This recommendation is based on the gradual decline in renin with age and the relative responsiveness of different ages of patient to the different classes of drug. However, there may be indications to use alternative agents as first-line therapy, such as the presence of proteinuria in patients with diabetes (suggesting the use of an ACE inhibitor) or prostatism in men (suggesting the use of an α blocker).

HOW COMMON ARE SIDE EFFECTS OF ANTI-HYPERTENSIVE MEDICATION?

Overall, side effects of anti-hypertensive medication are uncommon. Nevertheless, there are some well-documented side effects, such as cough with ACE inhibitors (approximately 10% of patients) or postural hypotension with α blockers. Patients should be warned of the more common side effects and also asked to read the patient information sheets that are now included within the packaging of all medications.

IS MONO-THERAPY OR COMBINATION THERAPY BETTER?

Clearly it is in everyone's interest if patients can be treated with as few drugs as possible. However, this is usually possible in only about a third of patients, and therefore two-thirds of patients are likely to require combination therapy.

- When using drugs in combination, the ABCD rule is helpful, in which A or B is combined with C or D (A, ACE inhibitor; B, β blocker; C, calcium channel blocker; D, diuretic; see Fig. 5.1).
- In terms of triple therapy, a commonly used regime is A + C + D (see http://www.bhsoc.org).

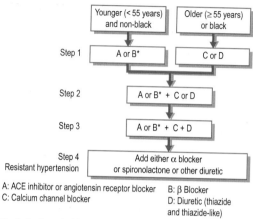

Fig. 5.1 The ABCD rule.

A: ACE inhibitor or angiotensin receptor blocker   B: β Blocker
C: Calcium channel blocker   D: Diuretic (thiazide and thiazide-like)

* Combination therapy involving B and D may induce more new-onset diabetes compared with other combination therapies

WHICH PATIENTS SHOULD BE REFERRED FOR SPECIALIST OPINIONS?

The following is a list of those patients with hypertension who should be considered for specialist referral.[1]

- Accelerated hypertension
- Severe hypertension (> 220/120 mmHg)
- Impending complications (e.g. transient ischaemic attack, left ventricular failure)
- Clue to a secondary cause in the history or examination (e.g. hypokalaemia suggesting possible Conn's syndrome)
- Renal impairment
- Proteinuria or haematuria
- Sudden onset or worsening of hypertension
- Resistance to multidrug therapy (three or more drugs)
- Young age of onset
- Multiple drug intolerances
- Multiple drug contra-indications
- Persistent poor compliance
- Labile blood pressure
- Possible white coat hypertension
- Hypertension in pregnancy

SHOULD ELDERLY PATIENTS WITH HYPERTENSION BE TREATED?

The benefits of treating older patients with hypertension are now firmly established. In particular, they are likely to get the same relative benefit as that of younger patients and—because they are at higher absolute risk of cardiovascular disease—have greater absolute benefit.

The same applies to patients with isolated systolic hypertension as to those with mixed systolic and diastolic hypertension. There is evidence of a reduction in morbidity, although not yet mortality, in patients over 80, and therefore treatment should not be withheld from the very elderly simply on the grounds of age.

WHEN IS 24-HOUR AMBULATORY BLOOD PRESSURE MONITORING USEFUL?

In the following groups, 24-hour ambulatory blood pressure monitoring is useful.

- Patients suspected of having white coat hypertension (e.g. marked blood pressure elevation in the absence of end-organ damage)
- Patients with particularly labile hypertension.
- Patients on anti-hypertensive therapy with symptoms suggestive of hypotensive episodes.
- It may also be useful in patients with apparent resistant hypertension to ensure that their condition is truly resistant to treatment and that they are not simply suffering from white coat hypertension.

It should be noted, however, that ambulatory blood pressure readings are generally 10–12/5–7 mmHg lower than those taken in the clinical setting, and this correction factor should be applied to translate the ambulatory values to clinic readings as a guide to therapy.

WHEN IS HOME BLOOD PRESSURE MONITORING USEFUL?

Home blood pressure monitoring can be used in the same situations as one would consider ambulatory blood pressure monitoring. It may also be helpful in speeding up diagnosis of hypertension and in assessing response to treatment, when the patients can be asked to return to the surgery with some readings taken in the home environment. Again, a correction factor of 10–12/5–7 mmHg should be added to home readings to translate them into clinic readings.

WHICH AUTOMATED SPHYGMOMANOMETERS HAVE BEEN VALIDATED?

Not all sphygmomanometers are accurate. In particular, aneroid devices are best avoided. Oscillometric and auscultatory devices can vary in the degree of accuracy, and the British Hypertension Society provides a list of approved devices available via the web site (http://www.bhsoc.org).

HOW OFTEN SHOULD PATIENTS BE REVIEWED?

In patients on treatment for hypertension who are at target in terms of blood pressure control, a review should be conducted every 6–12 months. In those who are not at target, the interval between visits will depend on the severity of hypertension and any existing co-morbidity. In general, such patients should be seen every 1–2 months and appropriate adjustments made to their therapy. Clearly, in patients with severe hypertension or severe coexisting disease, this interval may need to shortened considerably.

WHAT SHOULD BE DONE IF PATIENTS' BLOOD PRESSURE IS DIFFICULT TO CONTROL WITH DRUG THERAPY?

The most important thing is to confirm the diagnosis, and in this respect ambulatory blood pressure monitoring should be undertaken. A careful assessment of end-organ damage should also be performed and the patient's compliance with their medication should be assessed. With a modern armamentarium of medications, it is rare that truly compliant patients cannot achieve reasonable blood pressure control, although not all patients will achieve a target pressure of less than 140/85 mmHg.

WHICH PATIENTS SHOULD BE ADMITTED TO HOSPITAL FOR MANAGEMENT OF THEIR BLOOD PRESSURE?

Patients who require specialist investigation for secondary causes of hypertension may require hospital admission. Those with malignant hypertension or hypertensive emergencies, such as cerebral encephalopathy or hypertensive heart failure, require emergency admission. However, the vast majority of patients with hypertension can be treated as outpatients, either in general practice or secondary care.

REFERENCE

1. Williams B et al. British Hypertension Society guidelines for hypertension management 2004 (BHS-IV): summary. Br Med J 2004; 328: 634–640.

INDEX